BE
THE
FITTEST

Your ultimate 12-week guide to training smart, eating clever and learning to listen to your body

TYRONE BRENNAND

Photography by Martin Poole

QUADRILLE

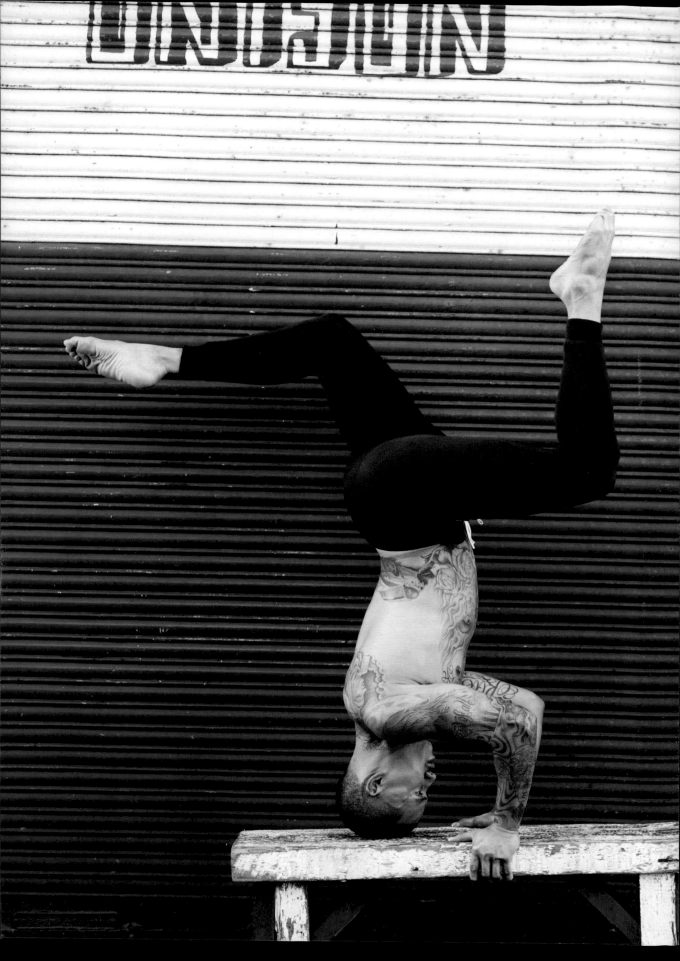

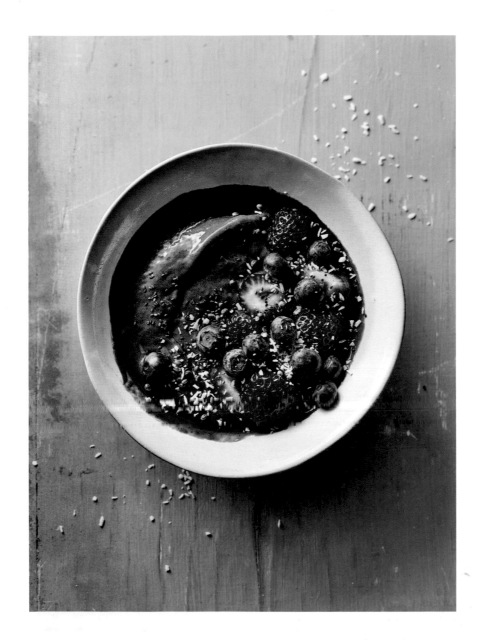

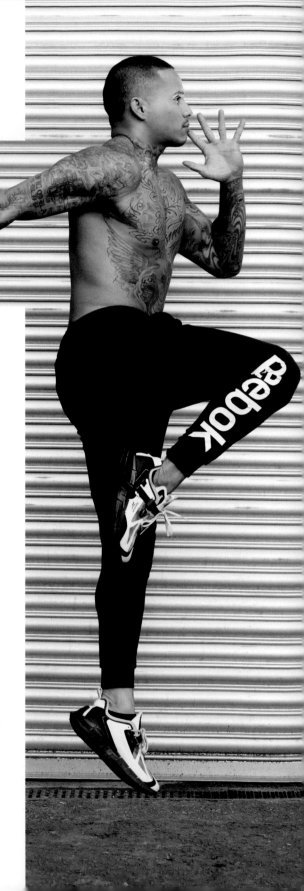

Medical disclaimer: The content of this book is for your general information and use only. Your use of any information is entirely at your own risk, for which neither the author nor the publisher shall be liable. It shall be your own responsibility to ensure that information in this book meets your specific requirements. Before taking part in any form of exercise, change of diet or consumption of a nutritional supplement you should always consult your doctor.

Publishing Director: Sarah Lavelle
Senior Commissioning Editor: Céline Hughes
Designer: Katherine Keeble
Photographer: Martin Poole
Food Stylist: Kim Morphew
Prop Stylist: Tamzin Ferdinando
Head of Production: Stephen Lang
Senior Production Controller: Nikolaus Ginelli

Published in 2020 by Quadrille,
an imprint of Hardie Grant Publishing

Quadrille
52–54 Southwark Street
London SE1 1UN
quadrille.com

Cataloguing in Publication Data: a catalogue record for this book is available from the British Library.

Text © Tyrone Brennand 2020
Design © Quadrille 2020
Photography © Martin Poole 2020

ISBN 978 1 78713 558 1

Printed in China

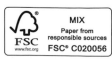

FSC
www.fsc.org

MIX
Paper from
responsible sources
FSC® C020056

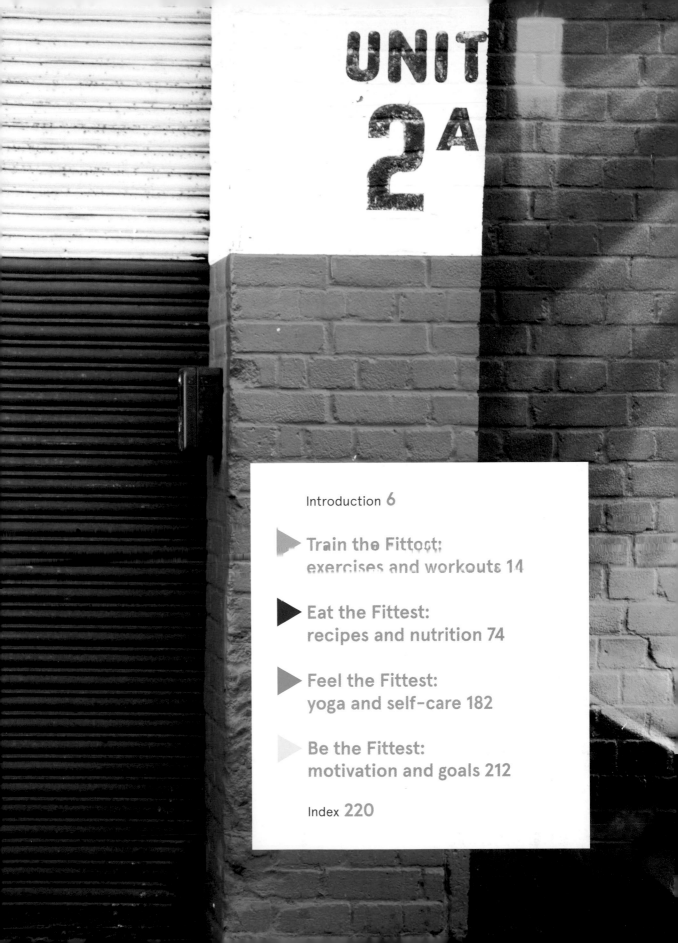

> **My teacher in Year 10 told me I would be a failure and that he would have the last laugh. My friend Nathan and I still talk about this and I use it as inspiration.**

My story

I have been interested in physical fitness for as long as I can remember. When I was about seven, I loved martial arts and was obsessed by reading martial arts and body building magazines. I would always try to copy Bruce Lee and other martial artists and the moves they did. I instantly gravitated towards the way they looked and was massively impressed by their physical presence. From then on, I became fascinated by the idea of pushing myself to achieve real results and to change my own body.

I grew up in London, living with my mum and sister. My mum had to work two jobs and money was very tight. I remember it as a time of eviction notices and having to ration food because we were struggling to pay the bills. It may sound tough, but at the time it was ok because I didn't know any different. I never knew my dad and I still don't know who he is, to this day. When I was 24, I found out that my sister was only my half-sister. This came as a real shock. Looking back at my childhood, my overall feeling about it is that it was fun, and I liked how things were, even though it wasn't the easiest.

At school I only really enjoyed doing sports and art. I remember going to my first gym class in school when I was around 13 years old. I wasn't particularly strong compared to some of the other kids that were in my school, but I really enjoyed it nonetheless. Another memory that sticks with me is that my teacher in Year 10 told me I would be a failure and that he would have the last laugh. My friend Nathan and I still talk about this and I use it as inspiration.

I left school with five GCSEs. At the time, I wanted to earn some money so I learnt how to cut Afro hair and started working in a barbershop on Sundays, while going to college during the week.

I remember skipping a lot of classes to go back to my house where I had made a home gym with a York bench and a few weights. Training was my real passion. After college, I went to art school but dropped out after only a few months.

I didn't have much guidance from my mum during this time, as she had lost her own mum (my grandmother), and had

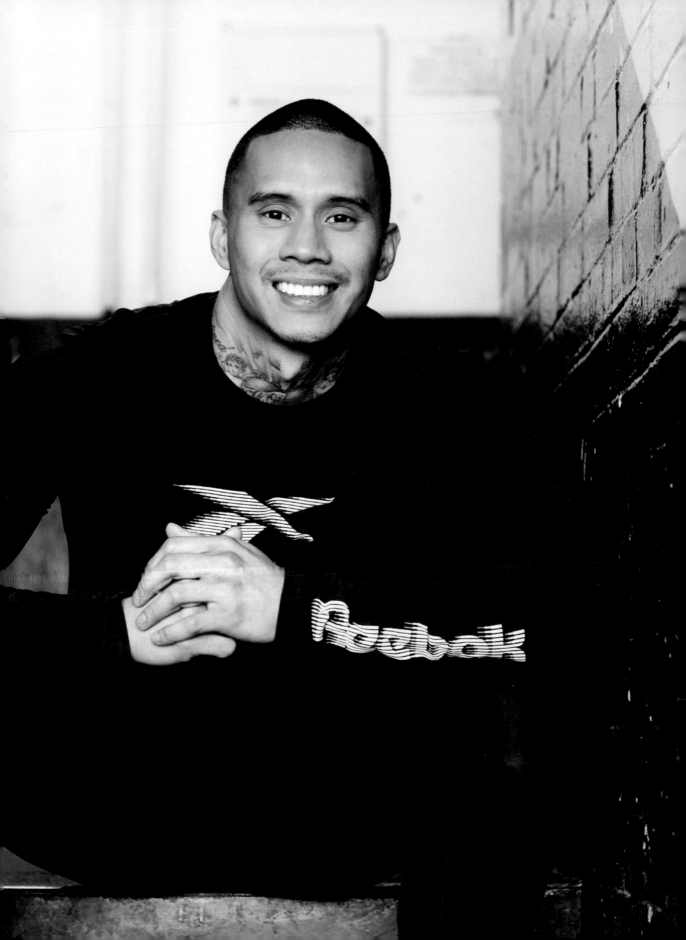

spent a lot of time abroad. My sister was at university, so I really didn't have anyone to answer to. I could just do what I liked. There were only really two things I wanted to do: to make money and to train. Growing up in London is weird – on one hand there is so much opportunity and on the other hand there is an immense amount of pressure from society, which brings with it doubt and fear of failure. It is also a city with a real mixture of rich and poor. A lot of my friends growing up were finding ways to make their own money, and not always by legitimate means. I was surrounded by this – I saw the glamorous side of money and the lifestyle it can bring but I also saw friends going in and out of prison and getting into life-threatening situations. I fell deeper and deeper into this lifestyle, and a few years later I found myself getting into a very bad situation. I was in the wrong place at the wrong time and ended up in serious trouble. My life changed in an instant, for the worse. I was in a really bad place. I was left with no hope, my life felt empty and the worst (and scariest) thing was that I didn't really care.

At this point, the things that really helped my mental health were exercise and training. I also had my first experience of yoga. I was given a book about it – I tried to read it but didn't really understand it. I was, however, drawn to the pictures and began to practise the moves that were shown.

At the same time, I started reflecting on things a lot and really wondered what I wanted to do with my life. I felt trapped in the world I had been living in. The only real passion I had (and my saving grace) was for training and exercise.

When I was 24, I found out that I was going to have my first child. That was what made me decide to make a conscious effort to start my own business. I didn't know what the business was going to be at that stage, as none of the little jobs I'd had working for other companies had really resonated with me. But I knew I had to change my life around.

Over the years I had been training with friends and lots of them had said I would make an amazing personal trainer. Not in a million years did I want to do that – at that time the typical personal trainer would work in a gym for a company and that just wasn't me. I did start to think about having a fitness blog, or a fitness video platform, but nothing really grabbed me at first. The thought of becoming a trainer kept on coming back to me and eventually I realized I could start my own personal training company and offer a unique service – and be better than anyone else out there!

I came up with a name for the business, Be the Fittest. From there, the journey really started. I knew I could leave my previous life behind. However, I didn't know how to start a business, nor did my mother or any of my friends. I had heard of The Prince's Trust, which helps young people with starting businesses, among other things. So I approached them and was able to go on a business starter's course. On completion of the course, I went away, built the business and ended up going on a panel interview with them, which I passed! They agreed to mentor and train me and I launched my business in 2014. I built a website and started promoting it. I literally had no clients and didn't really know where to start but I learnt about SEO (search engine optimization) through another Prince's Trust workshop and started implementing it into my website. It started to work. I then launched my Instagram account – initially just posting videos of me training the clients I had got through my website – and this brought in even more clients.

I became a Young Ambassador for The Prince's Trust in 2016 and now I am a part of board for their Rise campaign to raise money for young people. I attend events and speak to large audiences from the corporate world about my journey. I am also an ambassador for fitness brands Reebok and Grenade. I have an international online following, and am fully booked out with an amazing client base and a great team of trainers in London. I've trained clients for thousands and thousands of hours, at the same time spending time with my three kids and running my business. I am so proud of transforming so many people, while helping them to achieve their goals.

I have learnt so much from my clients, from all the struggles they have had and from every issue I was able to solve with them. I have now been given this amazing opportunity, to write a book and share all my knowledge with you. I hope that I can help each of you to achieve your goals. Together we will work out the best and most efficient way to get the results you want in the healthiest, smartest and fittest way.

Who is this book for?

This book is for anyone who wants to change their lives through health and wellness. For anyone who wants to take a more overall approach and make sustainable lifestyle adjustments.

You may not have any experience of training or have perhaps never stepped in a gym at all.

Or you may have had some experience in training and exercise – either way, this book will cater for you. There are three different levels: beginners, intermediate and advanced. Working your way through each section will allow you to build your strength, fitness and endurance.

Unlike a lot of fitness books, my book also includes information on the practice of yoga, breathing and meditation. The breathing exercises and meditation will help you to deal with stress, improving your clarity and strengthening your mental health. This works hand-in-hand with the exercise programme and will complement your physical training.

I hope that you will use this book as a tool for life. It will enable you not just to get through each day and to enjoy your fitness and exercise but also encourage you to work on different aspects that you would not normally work on through just normal exercise.

How to use this book

I want you to use this book like a personal tool. You can follow the programme step by-step, but you can also make this book your own. Take bits from it, add bits to it, use advice from all the different sections to improve on your own individual strengths and address your weaknesses.

You can expect this book to be fun, but also challenging. I want you to feel excited about using the book to identify something that you will be fully motivated and determined to achieve. This book will enable me to push you to the next level safely, but also according to your own level of fitness and strength. I will give you a whole programme, with three months of training, using over 150 different exercises. I will also teach you new training techniques, as well as using different techniques to relieve stress.

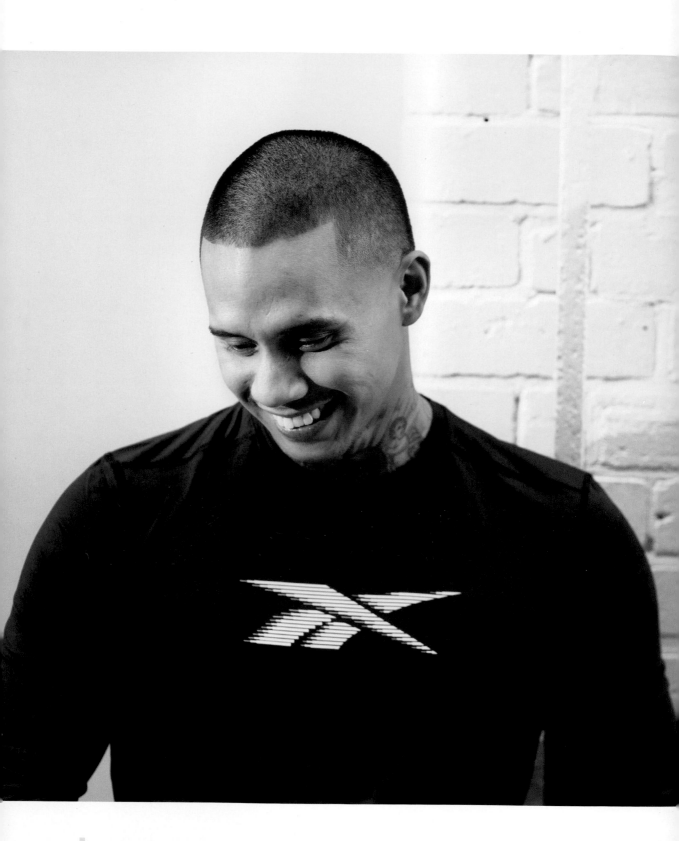

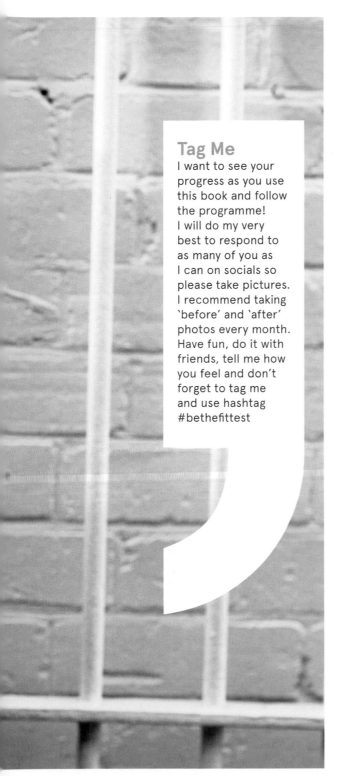

Tag Me

I want to see your progress as you use this book and follow the programme!
I will do my very best to respond to as many of you as I can on socials so please take pictures. I recommend taking 'before' and 'after' photos every month. Have fun, do it with friends, tell me how you feel and don't forget to tag me and use hashtag #bethefittest

Besides the physical training programme, I want you to think about your overall wellness. Read the sections on meditation and breathing and incorporate those into your daily life, particularly at times when you may feel stressed or anxious. Along with working on mental clarity through breathing and meditation, this book will also teach you the fundamentals of yoga and will show you many different yoga poses and stretches which you can do at home and incorporate into your own programme.

I have created a diet plan for you to follow, which should go hand-in-hand with your exercise programme to help you live the healthiest lifestyle possible. Following the plan will help you achieve your goals and give you the correct nutrients to exercise at your best level. As well as general rules and regulations to stick to, I have also given you over 60 recipes which have been created by me with input from head chef Scot Paterson and a dietician. What's great about these recipes is that you can buy these ingredients from any local store, each meal is simple and easy to make, but still tastes amazing and is of course packed with great nutrients. I would also encourage you to experiment and make the recipes your own, change the ingredients around to suit your own tastes.

I want this book to be something that you can come back to, and refer to, for many years.

What are YOUR goals?

Before you start the programme, answer the questions on the following page. This is a great way to really make your goals, and what you want to achieve, clear.

1 ▶ What are your dream goals?

2 ▶ What three things would you like to improve on over the next three months?

3 ▶ What have you been your main struggles in achieving goals?

4 ▶ Name two things which give you motivation.

5 ▶ What are your top strengths and your biggest weaknesses?

6 ▶ Are you willing to put in 100% effort to achieve your goals?

Make a note of your answers and refer back to them regularly during the training programme to keep your goals in mind and sustain your motivation. You might find that your goals evolve as you become stronger and fitter. See also page 218.

The 12-week programme

This is a 12-week programme, with a mixture of physical exercises focusing on my unique hybrid workout along with cardio exercise and strength work. This is balanced with exercises to improve your mental wellness such as meditation, breathing and yoga. There is also an Initiation for people who have never worked out or who are not quite ready to start the full 12-week programme.

Everyone is different, and every body is different. The results won't be exactly the same for everyone. However, what I can say, is that if you follow this programme, and stick to it as prescribed, then you will get stronger, fitter, lose body fat, get more toned muscles and feel better mentally and

physically, ultimately leading you to a happier and healthier life. From my experience, you will get out of it what you put in. As long as you stay dedicated and maintain consistency throughout the programme you will achieve results. Always keep this in mind!

Over the 12 weeks you will come across different types of disciplines, which will keep the programme varied and interesting:

▶ Cardio
▶ Strength training (upper and lower body)
▶ Calisthenics (exercises that rely on your own body weight)
▶ Fitness endurance
▶ Yoga
▶ Breathing
▶ Meditation

How does the programme work?

All the warm-ups, individual exercises and cool-down stretches are explained and illustrated on pages 19–52. Read them, try them out and familiarize yourself with them before you start your programme. Refer back to them whenever you need to in order to ensure that you're always doing the exercises with good form and technique.

Then the programme is broken down into phases.

The Testing Phase will help you to determine at which level you should start.

The Initiation is for total beginners and those who haven't exercised at all, who have suffered injuries or are coming back into training following a long break.

Then we have the main 12-week programme which is broken down into three phases: Beginner, Intermediate and Advanced.

Testing phase (page 54)

Initiation (page 54)

12-week programme (pages 68–73)
Beginner phase: Weeks 1–4
Intermediate phase: Weeks 5–8
Advanced phase: Weeks 9–12

Each day, throughout the programme, you will have specific workouts and tasks to complete. Each week there will be challenges and room for progress.

How to track your progress

Tracking your progress is very important. It's something I watch closely with all of my clients and it can provide motivation as well as more momentum. It will also help you to see if things are going along on the right path. You can track your progress in different ways:

Weight
If losing pounds is your goal, then jumping on the scales is a great way to see if you are getting results.

Pictures
Take 'before' pictures on your phone so that you have a visual comparison to look back at.

Performance
Noticing a difference in your performance each week during the exercise programme or improving on certain exercises is a great feeling and provides fantastic motivation. It's proof that you are getting fitter or stronger.

Clothing
Look out for differences in your clothing, for example, you may have lost some inches around your waist. Trying on a pair of jeans that you couldn't fit into before or even just looking at your outfit in the mirror and liking the way you look is definite progress.

Mood
Just waking up in the morning and feeling happier, healthier and better about yourself is progress. Having more energy which lasts throughout the day or just not feeling out of breath walking up the stairs as usual – these are great ways of knowing that the programme is working.

Tips before starting the programme

Remember throughout your journey the reason why you've started the programme, the end goal you desire, and know that you can do it! Everyone can achieve what they're aiming for. Just don't give up.

This is not a race, so take your time, make sure you do all the forms of exercise, meditation and yoga as best as you can.

Concentrate, give it 100%. Use your initiative, be smart and of course enjoy it and have fun.

It's not always simply about training harder, it's about training smarter and being wise. Listen to your body and don't overdo it. You will eventually achieve what you're trying to do but things don't happen overnight.

I post many of the exercises on my Instagram @bethefittest – check it out so you know you're doing everything correctly.

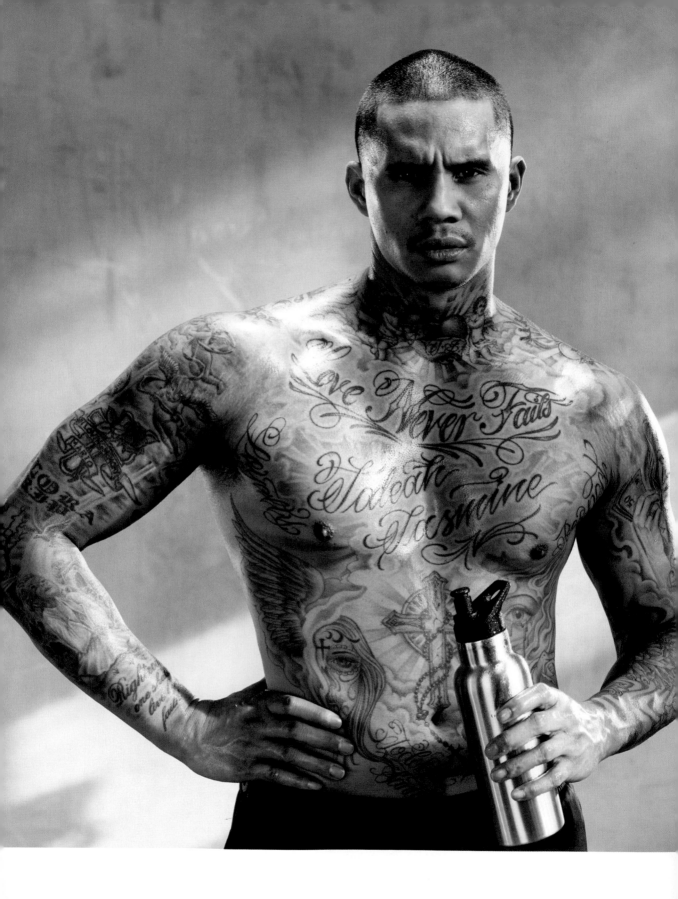

1

TRAIN THE FITTEST

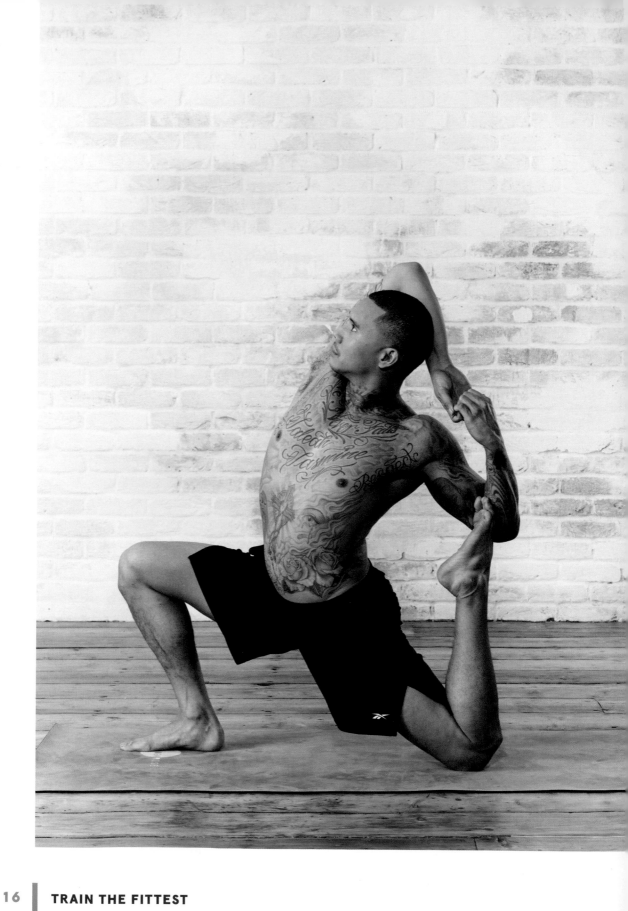

| **TRAIN THE FITTEST**

Throughout my years of training and helping clients reach their goals I've learnt that training and exercising can be daunting, especially if you haven't had much experience with it or you have never really enjoyed it.

I want to tell you all that **you can do this**. Some of my clients – see pages 66–67 – have achieved amazing results with no previous experience in exercise and previously no motivation. Some of them had never stepped foot in the gym or could hardly do even one squat. They had to start with the basics; we all have to start from somewhere and learn to take our time and do the homework! The one thing all the clients who achieve the best results have in common is perseverance both when training and sticking to the diet outside of exercising.

Always give 100% and the results will come. Take one day at a time; some days will feel amazing and others might feel super tough, but as long as you stay dedicated and consistent this is what counts. Every workout you complete brings you a step closer to achieving those goals you're striving for.

On those days when you feel like you can't exercise or you don't have any motivation, put on some good music, warm up properly and take your time. Think about your goals and how far you've come – then give it your best shot.

Remember, during exercise it's all about good technique and doing the exercises properly – don't rush them and do allow your muscles to burn! Regardless of your fitness level, just move your body, do it well and have fun.

You will have obstacles to overcome but every one of you can do this, no matter how hard it may seem. If everything was that easy, everybody would be the fittest, all the time! Be realistic and don't be too hard on yourself.

Let's change our lives for the better and get fitter, healthier, stronger and of course happier. ENEERRGGYY!

> You may feel frustrated, you may feel like you don't want to do it, like you might cry – but remember the reason you're doing it and what you set out to achieve.

BEFORE YOU START

Health warning

If you have any injuries or concerns about your health and physical fitness, it is imperative that you consult a doctor before starting to work out.

While you're exercising, if you experience any discomfort or pain, stop what you're doing immediately and seek medical advice.

Injury prevention tips

ALWAYS make sure you warm up the body before you start a workout. The muscles need to be eased into their hard work. If you're feeling particularly stiff, make sure you open up more during the warm-up. Do this by using a foam roller or trigger point ball to target areas that feel stiff or tight.

Similarly they need to be wound down slowly with stretching and a cool-down after a workout. Otherwise you will be much stiffer and more uncomfortable that you should be the following day. Stretching is so important in aiding recovery and reducing injury. When you train a lot in the week your muscles can get tight so you need to stretch them out. This will keep them supple and flexible enough to manage the full range of motion during exercise.

Use a foam roller and/or trigger point ball to help self massage and remove any knots in muscles on your days off.

During a workout, take your time to ensure that you're keeping good form and technique with each exercise. This will prevent injury and unnecessary discomfort and maximizes the good effects of the exercise.

What you'll need

Find somewhere to train where you're comfortable and have room to move around. If possible, put your mat on a hard surface so you can feel the floor through the mat. If you only have carpet, that's just fine.

You don't need any special kit to get started – a few essentials:

▶ Mat – make sure that it's thick and has good grip, like the ones made especially for yoga, to protect your knees and hands.
▶ Good workout shoes – they need to be stable and fit your feet well. Get advice in a shop or online about a type that's suitable for both working out and jogging, as these will have the right support for this programme and any other cardio work you do alongside it.
▶ Water.
▶ Yoga blocks – get two that look like bricks if you can, otherwise you can just use some thick books.
▶ Good music playlist (follow my Train the Fittest playlist on Spotify if you like!).
▶ Foam roller – not essential but great for recovery if you're exercising more than three to four times per week. It's great for self-massage and removing any tightness or knots in your muscles. It will prepare you well for your next workout session.
▶ Trigger point ball – again not essential but good for accessing those hard-to-reach and smaller areas that foam rollers can't reach.

Terms

▶ Rep = a repetition of a single exercise
▶ Set = several consecutive reps of a single exercise
▶ Round = a sequence of sets of different exercises

DYNAMIC STRETCH WARM-UPS

Forward leg kick

Begin standing, with your feet together, looking straight ahead. Put your hands on your waist. Kick one leg forward and backwards, with your foot flexed, trying to keep both legs as straight as possible, with the other foot firmly planted on the floor. Try not to move your upper body too much. Keep your core engaged and allow your hip flexors and hamstrings to stretch. Repeat on both sides.

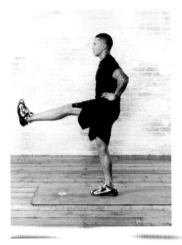 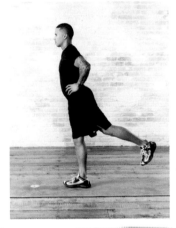

Lateral leg kick

Stand with your feet hip width apart. With your legs as straight as you can, lift one foot out to the side then kick your leg across your body in a lateral motion. Try and not twist your foot in the direction of the movement but keep the foot facing forward. Repeat for both sides.

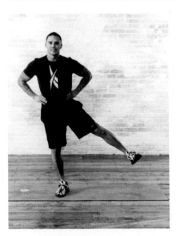 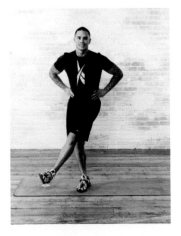

Walking high knee

Begin standing, with your feet hip width apart. Alternating them, one leg then the other, bring your knees up towards your stomach at walking tempo, keeping your back straight and chest open. Really try and drive the knee as high as you can, working the hip flexors and stretching out your glutes. Keep your arms bent and swing them backwards and forwards as if you were running, spreading your fingers out.

Walking heel to bum

Begin standing, with your feet hip width apart. Alternating them, one leg then the other, kick your heels to your bum, keeping your hands by your waist or on either side of your head, stretching out your quadriceps.

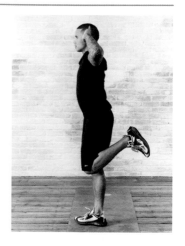

Hip rotation

Begin standing, with your feet hip width apart. Place your hands on your waist and make circular motions with your hips, allowing the circles to get bigger and bigger as your hips become more open. Change direction once you have completed one direction. Do 10–15 rotations on each side or until your hips feel looser and more stretched out.

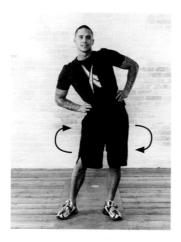 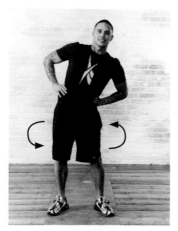

Forward and back arm circle

Begin standing, with your feet hip width apart. With your arms straight, rotate both arms forwards with a large circular motion 10 times and then bring them back the other way 10 times. Try to keep the upper body as still as you can to allow the shoulder to get a full rotation.

Bear hug

Stand with your feet hip width apart. Bring both arms out to your sides, with a slight bend at the elbow. Swing your arms forwards and backwards, in and out, stretching your chest and back. The motion should feel as if you're hugging a bear!

Lateral arm circle

Stand with your feet hip width apart. With both arms straight out to the sides laterally, move both hands round as if you were drawing a circle. Start off with small circles in one direction, increasing to bigger circles until you start to feel a burn in the shoulders, then repeat in the other direction.

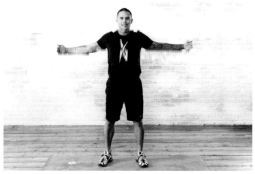

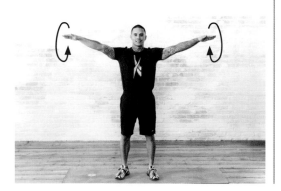

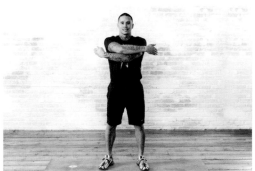

Floor wrist stretch

Start with your hands and knees on the floor, spreading your fingers out and keeping your arms straight. Looking towards the top of your mat, turn your left hand backwards so that the fingers are facing back towards your knees. Rock your body forwards and backwards while you hold your hand in position for a few seconds. Now twist back around so that the fingers are facing forwards and repeat with the other hand.

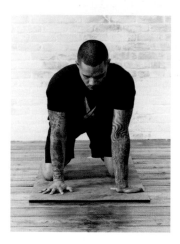 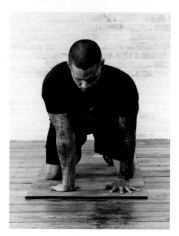

EXERCISES

Star jumps

Begin standing, with your feet together. Jump your legs in and out in a lateral movement, allowing your arms to follow. Keep your arms as straight as you can, moving in and out at a good tempo and allowing your heart rate to increase.

Squats on sofa or low chair

Begin standing in front of a sofa or low chair, with your feet hip width apart, keeping your core engaged and back straight. Keep your arms straight out in front of you. Squat down to sit on the sofa or chair then come back up to standing.

Squat

Begin standing, with your feet just past hip width apart. Slightly turn your toes out, keep your back straight and your core active. Start to stick your bottom out and bend at the knees. Suck your belly in and begin to bring your arms out in front of you. Open the chest and keep your back straight. Go as low as you can, depending on your flexibility and strength. Try to get your knees down to a 90-degree angle or a bit lower if you can. From the bottom of the squat, pushing through your glutes, hamstrings and core, lift your bum back up, straightening the legs back to standing. As you reach the top, squeeze your glutes together and then go back down for another rep as required.

Squat jumps on sofa or low chair

From standing and with your arms straight out in front of you, slowly sit down on either a sofa or low chair, keeping your back straight, legs active and core engaged. Push off through your legs (bring your arms down to your side), from sitting to standing, and as you reach standing position and your body is in a strong, balanced position, jump up into the air as high as you can and land softly with your feet firmly on the floor. If you can't jump, stand up as high as you can on your tiptoes instead. Go back down into the squat position, and repeat as required.

High level lunge

Start with your feet slightly apart. Move one foot forward about 4 steps in front of you so that your legs are split apart, one forward and one back. The back heel should be off the floor, resting on tiptoes. The front foot should be facing forwards. Bend the front leg 90 degrees, with the back leg as straight as possible. Lift your arms up straight in the air and hold. Your core should be engaged and back straight.

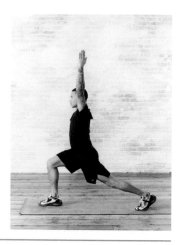

Press-up on knees

Start in a straight arm plank position (see right), hands just past shoulder width apart. With your knees on the floor, your feet up and starting with straight arms, slowly lower your chest to the floor. Keep your core engaged and back straight as you get to your lowest position. Look just past your hands. Push back up using your triceps and shoulders and exhaling.

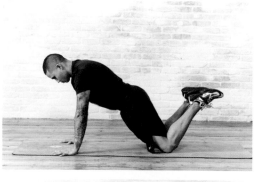

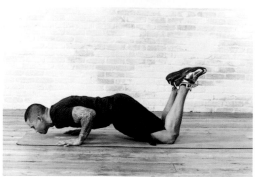

Straight arm plank

Lie on your front, with your feet together and hands flat on the floor directly under your shoulders. Push up with your whole body, so that your arms are straight, keeping your shoulders over your wrists. Protract your shoulders (rounding the upper back, moving your shoulders away from your spine) and tuck in your pelvis in a posterior tilt. Bring your knees off the floor keeping your legs straight so the only points of contact on the floor are your hands and toes. Look just past your hands. This is the 'straight arm plank position'.

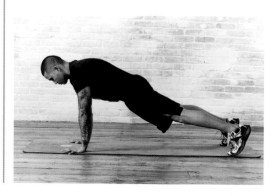

Plank press-up on knees

Start with your knees and hands on the floor. Keep the position of your hands shoulder width apart, protract your shoulders, keeping the shoulders over your wrists. Tuck in your pelvis in posterior tilt, then bring your right elbow and forearm to the floor. Bring your left elbow and forearm to the floor so you're in elbow plank position, then bring your right hand back up to where the elbow was, then the left, to come back into a straight arm plank. Your knees should be in the same position throughout. This is one repetition, leading through your right arm.

Walking mountain climber

Begin in a straight arm plank position (page 24), keeping your hands flat on the floor with your fingers spread out. With your arms straight, and shoulders over the wrists, protracting through the upper back (rounding the upper back, moving your shoulders away from your spine), tuck your tailbone in and bring one knee into the chest keeping the other leg straight. Alternate each leg, in and out.

Straight arm plank step-out

Begin in a straight arm plank position (page 24). Bring one leg out to the side and tap the toe down to the floor, then bring it back next to the other foot. Repeat with the other leg, alternating, and tapping each foot out one at a time.

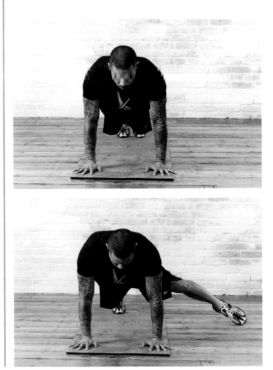

Downward facing dog

Begin with your hands and knees on the floor. Make sure your hands are flat on the floor and fingers are spread apart. Your knees should be below your hips and your toes should be tucked under. Pushing your hands against the floor, keeping your arms straight, lift your knees off the floor and gradually straighten your legs. Keep your heels up and toes on the ground, lengthening and lifting your tailbone towards the ceiling. Straighten your legs as much as you can while pushing away from the mat with your hands and arms. Draw your shoulders away from your ears and guide your heels towards the floor. Suck your belly in and keep lifting through your tailbone, breathe and stay here for the time needed.

Plank to downward facing dog

Start in a straight arm plank position (page 24), then pushing back through your arms, keeping your arms straight, lift your tailbone. Suck in your belly and allow your back to be straight, with your bum lifting to the ceiling.

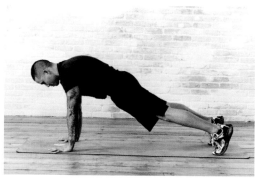

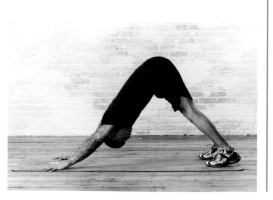

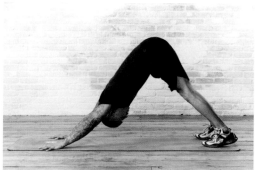

Walking burpee chest to floor

1 From a standing position, feet hip width apart, bend forward, bringing your hands flat on the floor. Step one leg back then the other, ending up in a plank pose.

2 Allow your whole body to come down to touch the floor.

3 Lift the torso up, step one leg forward, then the other. Coming up to standing, bring your hands into the air above your head and then jump up as high as you can. Repeat, alternating the leading leg.

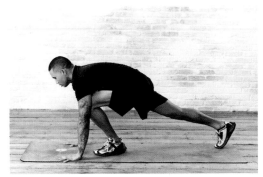

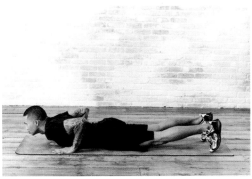

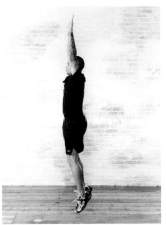

Elbow plank

Lie on your front, with your feet together and your elbows under your shoulders with your hands on the floor in front of you, clasped together. Lift up through the knees, keeping the legs active and rounding your upper back, protracting the shoulders. Keep your stomach tight and your bum down, holding the plank position.

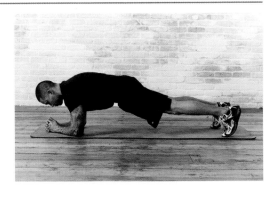

Slow glute kick pulse

1 With your hands and knees on the floor, keeping your shoulders over your wrists, extend one leg out straight behind you, pointing the toe, keeping the other knee on the floor.

2 Keeping your hips square, pulse the extended leg up and down with control, slowly contracting through the glutes.

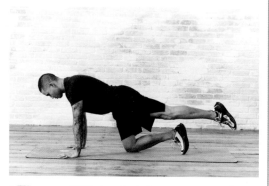

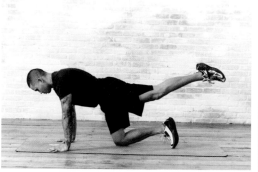

Slow donkey kick

With your hands and knees on the floor, and your shoulders over the wrists, keep one knee on the floor while lifting the other leg up into the air. Keep the leg bent and the foot flexed. Bring the knee down towards the floor and then kick it back out, keeping the leg bent. Squeeze through the glute muscles.

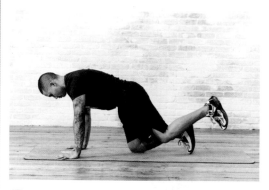

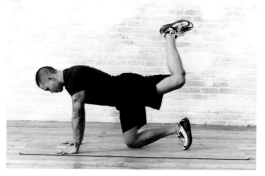

Sumo squat

Starting from standing, point your toes out and bring your feet just past hip width apart. As you come down into a squat, bring the knees out in line with your feet, keeping your back straight, chest open and holding when your knees are at 90 degrees. Hold for your desired time then come back up to standing position.

Static lunge

From standing, feet slightly apart and your hands on your waist (or out to the side for easier balance or – for extra support – on the knee you're about to bring forward), bring one leg forward and the other leg back, with the back heel off the floor. Keep the front leg bent and the back leg straight, with the hips square. Bring the back knee down towards the floor, keeping the front leg bent, and then come back up slowly and in a controlled manner.

Reverse leg raise

1 Lie down on the floor on your back and bring both legs up straight into the air, keeping your feet together.

2 Slowly start bringing one leg down towards the floor, keeping the other leg up in the air, as straight as you can.

3 As the leg comes down towards the floor don't let it touch the floor, keep it 2–3cm (¾–1¼in) off the ground, then bring it back up towards the other leg. Repeat on other side for the desired reps.

Malasana stretch hold

Starting from standing, point your toes out and bring your feet just past hip width apart. Come down into your lowest squat, then bring your elbows inside of your knees and allow your hips to drop as low as they can, keeping your back straight and your chest open. Stay here and breathe and slowly allow the hips to open. Push out through the elbows against your knees, stretching through your groin and legs.

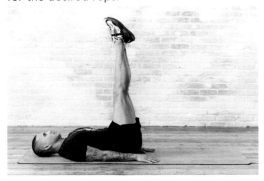

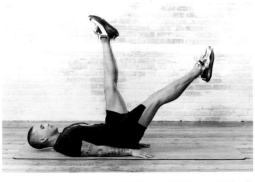

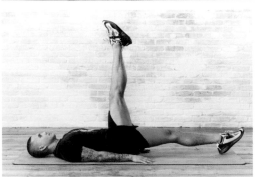

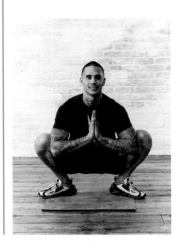

Squat floor touches

From standing, feet hip width apart and toes slightly pointing out, bend at the legs, bringing the bum down towards the floor. Look straight ahead. Keep your back straight as you go down into a squat position, touching down onto the floor with one hand, and then standing back up. Repeat this, alternating the hands as you come down.

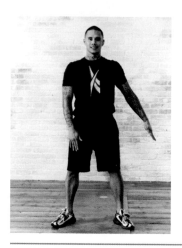 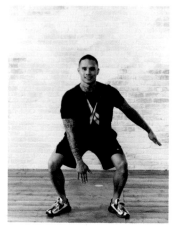 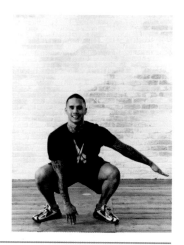

Squat hold on wall

Stand against a clear bit of wall and, feet hip width apart, lower down into a squat position keeping your back flat against the wall. Place your hands by your head, fingertips to your ears, and bring your elbows back allowing them to touch the wall. Ideally your knees should be at a 90-degree angle, keeping all the tension in the legs and glutes. Remain in position for the time required.

Leg raise and butt lift

Lie down on the floor, hands underneath your bum, and follow the same protocol as for a normal leg raise (page 34), but as your feet and legs reach up to 90 degrees, raise your bum into the air, squeezing and contracting the glutes. Try to make sure the legs stay vertical and are not coming down towards your head as you lift up. Bring your bum back down towards the floor in a slow and controlled way, then bring your legs back down to finish.

Knee raise

1 Lie down on the floor on your back with your feet and knees together, place your hands underneath your bum and bring your feet off the floor by a few inches, squeezing your legs together and keeping them straight.

2 Bring your knees in towards the chest as far as you can, keeping your feet and knees together and squeezing your core, then slowly straighten your legs and bring your feet back down towards the floor, keeping them a few inches off the floor. If you have a sore back, you can lower the feet until the heels touch the floor. Repeat as required.

Boat pose

Sit on your mat with your legs out in front of you. Balance on your sit bones, so that your feet are off the floor, as well as your upper back and lower back. Keep your back as straight as you can. Either bend your legs or keep them straight depending on your strength. Keep your hands and arms out in front of you for balance and hold the tension in your core.

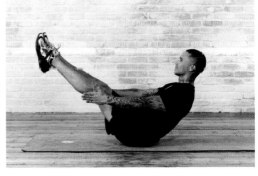

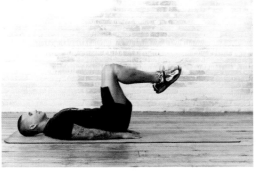

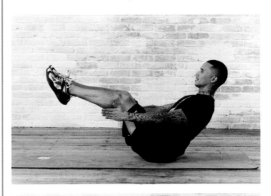

Jogging high knee

Jog on the spot, pumping each of your knees up towards your chest in turn. Pump your arms at the same time.

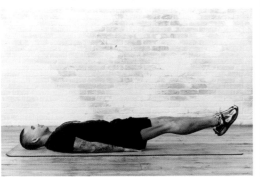

Straight arm walk-out

Start from standing. Bending your legs, bring your hands down towards the floor. Keeping your arms straight, from here walk your hands out forwards until you get to a straight arm plank position (page 24), then walk your hands back, bending your legs and coming up to standing.

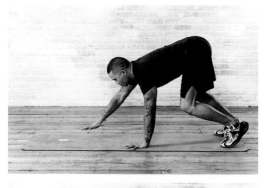

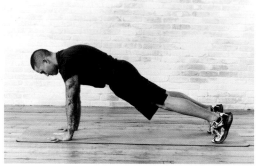

Controlled negative full press-up

Start in a straight arm plank position (page 24), hands just past shoulder width apart, then slowly bring the whole body down towards the floor, head always in front of your shoulders and chin slightly up. Try not to look down or drop your chin to your chest. Make sure you are controlling every single part of the movement until your body reaches the floor. Try not to allow your hips to dip down towards the floor, keep looking just above the space between your hands. Once you reach the floor, come back up to press-up position any way you want to.

Tricep press-up on knees

Start in a straight arm plank position (page 24). Bring in your hands slightly closer together so that they're within shoulder width apart. With your knees on the floor, and feet together and lifted, slowly come down, bringing your chest towards the floor. Your elbows should be tucked in. Keep control through every step of the motion. As you reach the lowest point, contract through the core and push out through your arms, shoulders and chest until you come back up to the straight arm plank position.

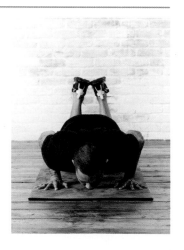

Downward facing dog, knee to tricep touch

1 Start from downward facing dog position (page 26). Lift one leg up into the air, keeping both legs straight.

2 Leaning forwards, start to bring the shoulders over the wrists, bringing your bum down. Slowly bring one knee towards your elbow. As you lean forward more, bringing the shoulders over the wrists, bring the knee into the elbow and allow it to touch, or bring it as far forward as you can. Once it touches, or you get to your furthest point, then push back through your hands and arms and bring the leg back into the air. Repeat on the other side.

Corkscrew

1 Start in a downward facing dog (page 26). Lift one leg into the air, keeping both legs straight.

2 Lean forward, bringing the bum down. Bring the knee of the raised leg towards your chest.

3 Bring the opposite hand off the floor and lift it straight up towards the ceiling, while kicking the opposite leg through in a side plank. Bring the arm and leg back into a down dog position. Repeat on the other side.

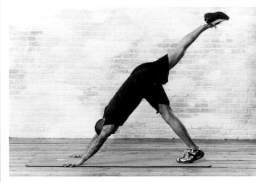

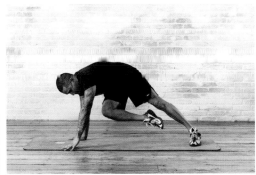

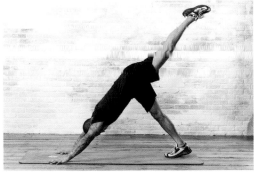

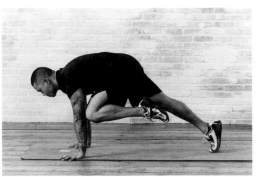

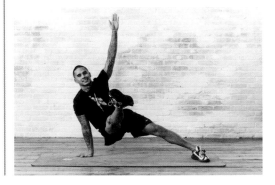

Elbow plank hip dip

1 Start in elbow plank position (page 27). Resting on your elbows with your hands clasped on the floor, keep your shoulders protracted and tuck in your tailbone.

2 With your legs active and your toes tucked in, dip one hip down towards the floor, keeping your core engaged. Bring the hip back around, then dip the other hip towards the floor and repeat the movement.

Elbow side plank

Start off in elbow plank position (page 27), then begin to turn to your side, stacking one foot on top of the other, while continuing to twist onto your side. Bring one elbow off the floor so you're balancing on the other elbow. Place the other hand either on your waist or straight up in the air. Place one foot on top of the other, or separate the feet. For a harder varation, lift the top leg into the air. Hold for the desired time.

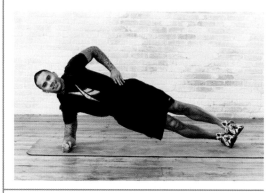

Leg raise

Lie down flat on the floor with your hands underneath your bum, feet and knees together. Keeping your legs as straight as you can, slowly lift both feet off the floor, bringing your legs up to a 90-degree angle. If at any time your back starts to hurt, you can bend your knees. Either way, keep your legs in one position – straight or bent – and do not change them. Slowly bring them back down towards the floor, keeping your legs in the same position that works for you and your core engaged as you reach back down. Lift your legs up and down for the amount of reps required.

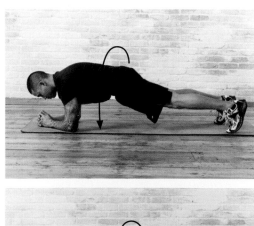

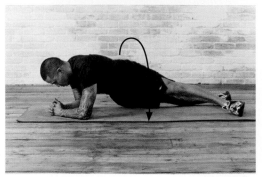

Single leg knee to chest

1 Lie down on your back with your legs flat on the floor and hands over your head.

2 With momentum, bring your hands off the floor, pushing your upper back off the floor and at the same time bring one knee in towards your chest and touch your foot. Come back down to the starting position, then, pushing all the way back up through your arms, bring the opposite knee in towards your chest and alternate the knees for every rep.

Scissors

Lie down flat on the floor with your hands underneath your bum, feet together. Lift your head off the mat and look towards your feet. Lift your feet about 8cm (3in) off the floor, then, moving your feet up and down slowly, bring the feet apart, separating them by around 50cm (20in). Each rep is when you bring one leg up and the other leg down.

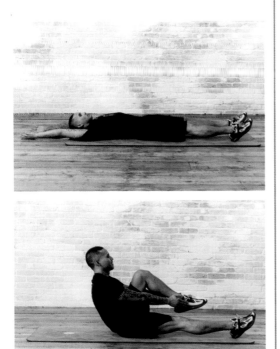

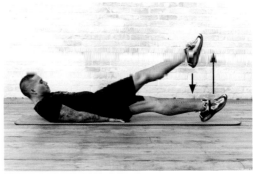

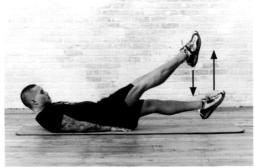

Flutters

This is very similar to the scissors (page 35). Instead of bringing one leg up and one leg down, bring one leg over to the side and the other leg under, to the opposite side. Then change over, bringing the top leg back down and across and bringing the bottom leg up and back around in the opposite direction.

Back extension

Lie down on your front, either placing your hands by your head, or for a harder variation with your arms straight out in front of you. Lift your arms, chest, lower thighs and knees off the floor and squeeze in for half a second at the top of the rep then bring both the upper body and legs back down towards the floor, then come back up for another rep.

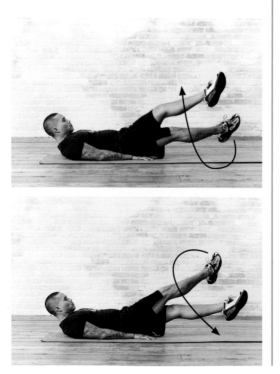

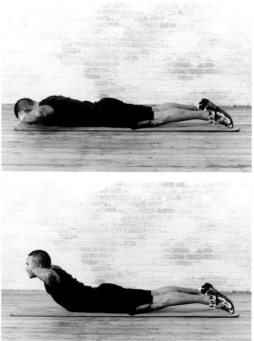

Arch

Lie down on your front, with your arms straight out in front of you, and your legs straight, pointing your toes. Lift as high as you can through your arms, lifting the chest and lifting through your legs, with your thighs off the floor. Hold as high as you can for the specified time.

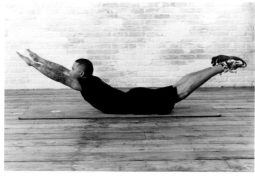

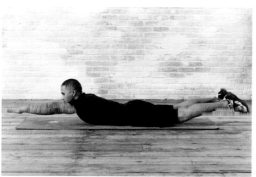

Forward lunge

Start with your feet slightly apart. Put your hands on your waist (or out to the side for easier balance or – for extra support – on the knee you're about to bring forward). Move one foot forward about 4 steps in front of you and then, bending both legs, bring your back knee down towards the floor as far as you can with the front leg at a 90-degree angle. Push up through your front leg as you come back up. Step the front leg back. Repeat with the same leg for the required number of reps.
*Alternating forward lunges - alternate the legs for the required number of reps instead of doing all the reps on the same leg.

Full press-up

Begin in straight arm plank position (page 24). Bring the hands just past shoulder width apart. From here, making sure the whole body is active, start bringing the chest towards the floor. Make sure the shoulders stay over the wrists, keeping your head slightly up. The bum should be neither dropping towards the floor or too high up into the air. When you get to the lowest point squeeze your muscles and push through your arms and chest to come back up to your starting position. Do this again for the amount of reps required.

Reverse lunge

This is similar to the forward lunge above but instead of bringing the leg forward to start the repetition, you step the leg backwards. Bring the leg backwards and bring the knee down towards the floor, with the front leg bent at a 90-degree angle. Push off through the front leg and bring the back leg back to standing position. Repeat with the same leg for the required number of reps.
*Alternating reverse lunges – alternate the legs for the required number of reps instead of doing all the reps on the same leg.

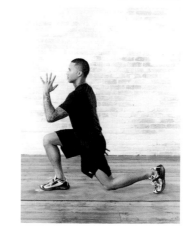

Side lunge

From standing, feet together, hands on hips, step out to the side as wide as you can. Move your weight slightly over to the side you have stepped out on, keeping that knee bent and the other leg straight. Both feet should be flat on the floor. Lunge and go deeper into the bent leg and then from the deepest position, push up and away, back to standing position. Keep your back straight and core engaged. Repeat with the same leg for the required number of reps.
Alternating side lunges – alternate the legs for the required number of reps instead of doing all the reps on the same leg.

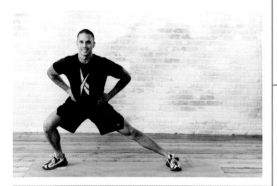

Snap jump

Start in a straight arm plank position (page 24). Keep the shoulders forward and either jump the feet out and then back, or walk them forward and back. Or for the harder variation jump the feet forwards to about 15cm (6in) behind the hands, bringing the bum in the air, and then back to plank.

Crunch

Lie down on your back. Either place your feet flat on the floor, knees bent, or bring your feet into the air and cross your legs. From here, place your hands by your head (fingertips by ears and elbows out to the side) and lifting through your core, bring your upper back off the floor. Contract the core, squeezing for half a second, then slowly come back down. Repeat as required. If you start getting any pain in the neck, take a rest until the pain is relieved then carry on.

Sit up

Lie down on your back. Place your feet flat on the floor with your knees bent. Place your hands up over your head, and using the momentum of your arms, push up and lift the upper back off the floor, bringing your chest towards your knees. If you struggle with bringing your chest all the way to the knees, then place your legs flat on the floor and do your sit ups in this position. If you are still struggling, just crunch up as high as you can and keep on doing the repetitions. Over time, you will become strong enough to do the full sit up.

Reverse plank

Start in a seated position with legs straight out in front of you. If you struggle, keep your knees bent. Place your hands either side of your bum with your arms straight, palms flat on the floor, with your fingers facing forward towards your feet. Start lifting up through the hips, straightening out your legs, and try to bring your feet flat on the floor. Lift up and open through the chest. Keep lifting the hips towards the ceiling, keeping your head in a neutral position looking up towards the ceiling.

High level lunge pulse

With one foot in front of the other in a static lunge position (page 28), bring your hands over your head, keeping your arms as straight as you can, or place your hands on the front knee for support, or place them on your waist. From here, bring the knee down as low as you can towards the floor and then back up. Keep going up and down in a pulsing motion for the amount of reps or time required.

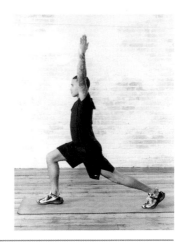

Shoulder taps

Start in a straight arm plank position (page 24). Keeping the core engaged, and taking care not to dip the hips from side-to-side, bring one hand up to tap the opposite shoulder. Bring the hand back down to the floor then alternate the hands, doing the same on the other side.

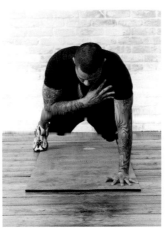

One leg straight arm plank

Start in straight arm plank position (page 24). Keeping your whole body and legs active, making sure your shoulders are protracted, slowly bring one leg off the floor as high as you can, balancing on one leg and keeping both legs as straight as you can. Try to not curve the back and hips sideways, keeping as straight as you can.

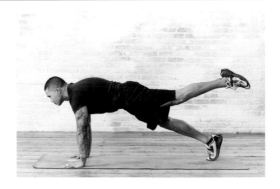

Burpee chest to floor

Follow the description of the walking burpee chest to floor on page 27 but jump your feet back from standing rather than stepping it back in, then when your chest is to the floor, straighten your arms to raise yourself back up to plank position, then jump your feet back in. Then once both feet are on the floor, jump with hands up in the air, as high as you can. Make sure to keep your back straight throughout, especially while jumping and stepping in and back.

Running high knee

Run on the spot – faster and harder than you would for jogging high knees on page 31 – bringing the knees as high as you can. Keep your back straight and chest open, pumping the arms as you're running.

Flip the dog

1 Starting from straight arm plank position (page 24) go into your straight arm side plank (page 42), with one hand on the floor and the other hand on your waist or up in the air. For a harder variation at this point, lift the higher leg up into the air.

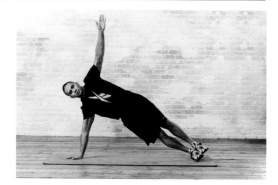

2 Step the top higher leg behind you so that that both feet are apart on the floor. Open through your hips, pushing through your legs and bringing your hips as high as you can. Bring the hand which is not on the floor down towards the floor, opening your chest to the ceiling.

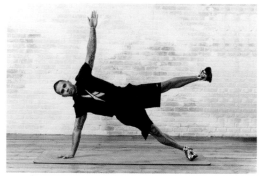

3 Stay here at your most open position for the required time, then flip your leg back around to your plank pose, bringing both hands back down to the floor.

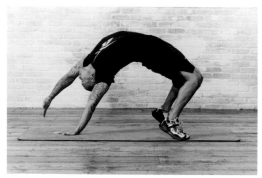

Elbow plank pike walk-in

Start in an elbow plank position (page 27) with your hands flat on the floor. Your elbows should be shoulder width apart, with your hands slightly closer together, with around a hand space in between. Slowly walk your feet in, taking small steps towards your elbows, bringing your feet as close as you can, raising your bum in the air. Either stay here and hold, or walk the feet back down, coming back towards plank position.

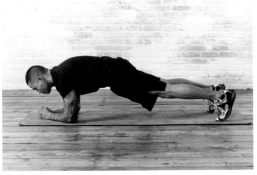 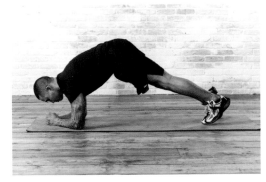

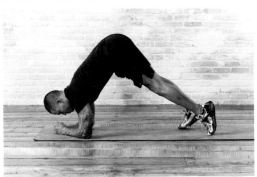 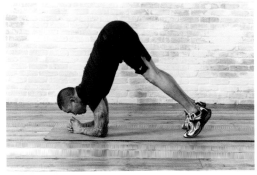

Low squats

Start in the same position as a normal squat (page 23), but as you come down allow your hips and bum to go down to their lowest point, trying to get a full range of motion. Keep your back straight, chest open and core engaged. As you reach the bottom of the squat, push through your glutes, your quads and your hamstrings, keeping your back straight all the way up to standing position. Squeeze the glutes at the top. Repeat for the required amount of reps.

Squat holds

Start in your squat position (page 23) and come down in exactly the same way. As you reach the bottom of your squat, hold in this position, keeping your whole body engaged – your core and your stomach tight, shoulders back, chest open and back straight, allowing all of the contraction and muscle work in the legs. Hold for the desired time, then come back up to standing position.

Straight arm walk-out with alternating knee drive jump

1 Start from standing. Bending your legs, bring your hands down towards the floor. Keeping your arms straight, from here walk your hands out forwards until you get to a straight arm plank position (page 24), then walk your hands back, bending your legs and coming up to standing.

2 Bring your knee up into the air and drive it up into the air, jumping up at the same time.

3 For a harder variation (bottom picture, below), when you start Step 1 above, keep one leg on the floor and one in the air. When you walk your hands back, automatically come up and drive the knee of the leg that's not on the floor up towards the chest. Come back down then change over to the other side.

Straight arm side plank

Lie on your side with your legs straight and feet together, and your lower hand below the corresponding shoulder. Raise your other arm up straight up in the air or rest your hand on your waist. Push your lower hand down and lift yourself up off the mat, straightening your arm, lifting your hips off the floor and keeping your knees on the floor. Hold here for the desired duration.

*Harder variation (picture below) – lift your hips up and straighten your lower arm as in the picture. Either stacking one foot on top of the other or bringing one foot in front of the other, place your hand flat down onto the floor, facing forwards, and keeping your arms straight, lift the hips off the floor, as high as you can. Lift the top leg up and bring back down.

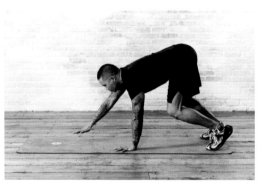

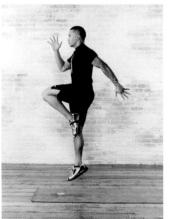

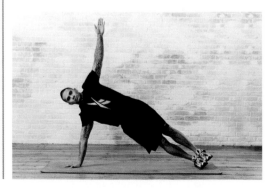

Side elbow plank hip dip

1 Start in a elbow side plank position (page 34), lift your hips as high as you can, then slowly start bringing the bottom hip down towards the floor.

2 Try to bring the hip as close to the floor as possible and then bring the hip back up. Every time the hip goes towards the floor this counts as one rep. Repeat as required on the other side.

Squat jump

Start in the squat position (page 23) with your arms straight out in front of you, and go down into your squat. As you come up, push through the legs, bring your arms down to your side and as you almost get to standing, carry the movement on and jump up, straightening the body. As your feet touch back down to the floor allow your muscles to take control and go back down into the squat. Keep on repeating this movement. Every time you do a jump you count this as one rep.

Squat jump touchdown

This is very similar to the normal squat (page 23), but instead of keeping your arms up as you come down into the squat, one hand comes down towards the floor as you squat down. As soon as you touch the floor, extend through your legs, keeping your body as straight as you can, jumping up into the air. As your feet touch down, alternate the hands. The other hand will come down and touch the floor. Repeat this movement for the required amount of reps.

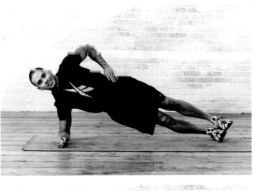

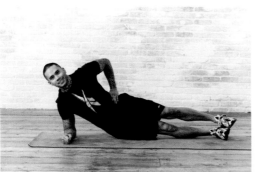

Plank press-up

Starting in a straight arm plank position (page 24), bring your right elbow and forearm down to the floor, keeping your hips as square as you can. Drop the left elbow and forearm down to the floor. Now you will be in an elbow plank position (page 27). Bringing your right hand back up to where your elbow was, push through the arms and bring your left hand back to where the left elbow was, ending up back in your straight arm plank. Do this for the required reps and change over, leading with the other arm first.

Lateral touchdown run

Using your mat as a guide, run in side steps across the mat keeping your feet facing forwards. Touch down on the floor with one hand once you reach the edge of your mat then run back across to the other side. Make sure you keep your back straight. Each time you touch down it is one repetition.

One leg handstand jumps

1 Start off in downward facing dog position (page 26), then bring one leg up into the air. Bend the knee of the leg that's on the floor and push off on that leg to jump both feet off the floor.

2 Keeping the shoulders forwards, bring your bum up into the air and aim to straighten one leg while the other is halfway up – this is airtime, where you're only touching the floor with your hands. Then bring the leg closest to the floor back down, leaving the other leg lifted in the air. Repeat for the required number of reps.

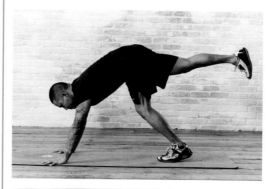

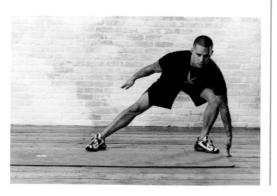

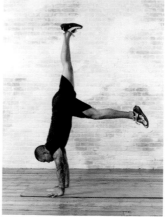

Full wheel

1 Lie on your back, arms by your sides, knees above your heels, feet parallel and hip width apart. Lift your bum in the air and push through your hips using your legs. Interlace your fingers under your bum and straighten your arms. Wiggle your shoulders to open up the chest as much as you can, keep pushing your hips up. Stay here for 5 breaths then come down to the mat and relax. This is a warm-up for the full wheel.

2 Bring your hands behind your ears, inverting your hands down towards the floor and elbows to the ceiling. Initially lift through your hips first, just a couple of inches and then slowly lift your shoulder blades and sacrum simultaneously to press straight up, also using your legs to help push up. Now extend and push up through your arms, trying to get them straight, moving towards achieving a 180-degree angle in your shoulders. Keep your arms and legs parallel to each other. Try to turn your triceps towards your face to maintain the external rotation in your arms and keep pushing from your legs towards your arms to open through your shoulders and chest.

3 Stay here for the required amount of time, then slowly come down, bringing your chin in to your chest as you come down. Lie down and prepare to come up one more time.

V up

Start from lying down on the floor with your hands over your head and legs straight. Lift up through the upper back, hands off the floor, then bring the legs up at the same time. Either keep your legs straight or have them bent. Bring your hands up towards your shins, touching them, and slowly come back down. Keep the body symmetrical through every part of the movement.

Straight arm plank rock

Starting from a straight arm plank position (page 24), making sure you're protracting through the upper back, tucking the tailbone in, with your legs active. Rock forwards and backwards, bringing your shoulders over your wrists, spreading your fingers out, with your hands flat on the floor, making sure you can feel the muscles in your shoulders working.

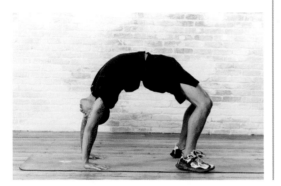

Diamond press-up

Either do these from full press-up position keeping your knees off the floor, or place your knees on the floor. Place your hands in a diamond position flat on the floor – thumbs and index fingers together, creating a diamond shape. Start to bend your arms and bring the chest towards the floor, letting your elbows come out to the side and keeping the shoulders over the wrists. When you get to the lowest point, push up using your triceps, core and shoulders back to the starting position.

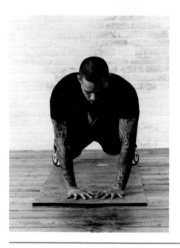 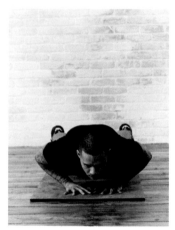

Half press-up hold

Begin in straight arm plank position (page 24), your hands just wider than shoulder width apart. Start off either with your knees on the floor or – for a full variation, with the knees off the floor – keeping your hands just past shoulder width apart as you come down, bring your chest towards the floor in the press-up position. Go to your lowest point and hold that position for the amount of time required. Make sure you keep the whole body engaged. Squeeze every muscle to hold yourself in place.

Sumo squat jumps

Follow the same protocol as for the sumo squat (page 28), and as you come down to the bottom of the sumo squat and you push up to where you're about to stand, jump up at the top of the rep trying to get as much air and power through the jump as possible. As the feet land back down on the floor, smoothly come back down into the lowest position of the sumo squat and keep on repeating for the required amount of reps.

Tricep press-up and single arm raise

1 Start in straight arm plank position (page 24). Drop your knees to the floor, place your hands on the floor within shoulder width apart. As you bring your chest towards the floor, keep your elbows tucked in so that you are working your triceps. If you're strong enough, you can do this press-up without the knees on the floor.

2 As you push back up from your deepest point, when your arms are straight bring your knees off the floor so you are in a straight arm plank position. From here, raise one arm up straight in front of you, as high as you can, keeping the arm straight. Then bring the arm back down to your straight arm plank pose, dropping the knees back down. Repeat the press-up, coming up and lifting the other arm.

Pincha single leg hold

1 Start in a downward facing dog position (page 26). Bring your elbows and forearms to the floor. Keep your hands flat on the floor but bring them in towards each other, keeping them one hand apart.

2 Walk your feet in towards your elbows, keeping the bum up high in the air, as far as you can go. Then lift one leg into the air. Holding this position, keep the shoulders forward and your core engaged, push through your shoulders and arms away from the floor. Hold the leg in position for the required time, changing legs if prescribed.

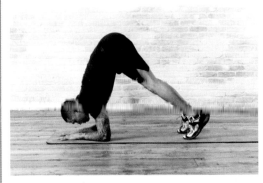

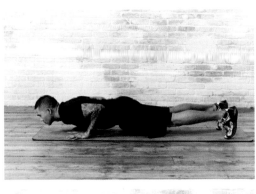

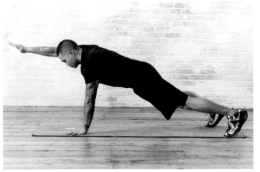

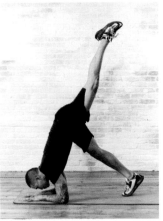

Boat pose scissors

Start off in a boat pose position (page 31) with your feet and upper back off the floor so you're balancing on your sit bones. Either place your hands behind your back flat on the floor or bring them up by your chest. Move one leg up and the other down, in turn. Remain in a balanced position, making sure you're keeping your core engaged and squeezing your abs.

Boat pose flutters

Start off in a boat pose position (page 31) with your feet and upper back off the floor so you're balancing on your sit bones. Either place your hands behind your back flat on the floor or bring them up by your chest. Bring one leg over the other, squeezing your legs in opposite directions, then reverse the movement, bringing the bottom leg over the top, and the top leg underneath the bottom. Repeat for the amount of reps required.

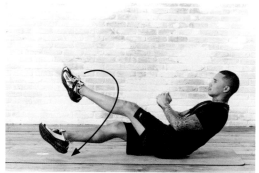

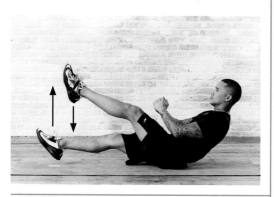

Squat pulse

Standing, with your feet hip width apart, come down into a squat position. As you reach down, when your knees are at a 90-degree angle or just past it, hold this position then slowly bring your bum a bit higher, so your knees are bent just above 90 degrees. As soon as you get there, bring it back down low and bounce/pulse up and down in a controlled movement, allowing the legs to burn.

Make sure you keep your back straight and chest open.

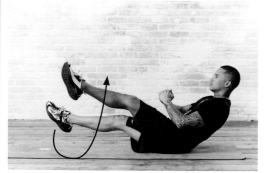

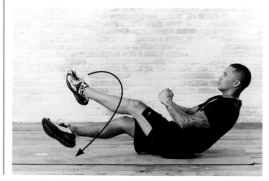

Boat pose pulses

Start off in a boat pose position (page 31) with your feet and upper back off the floor so you're balancing on your sit bones. Either place your hands behind your back flat on the floor or bring them up by your chest. Keeping your feet together, pulse your knees in towards your chest, then bring them back to the starting position. Keep on pulsing in and out, making sure you keep your back straight and your core engaged, squeezing through each contraction.

Low boat pose

Start off in a boat pose position (page 31), bringing your feet off the floor, with your legs either bent or straight, keeping your back straight and upper back off the floor, balancing on your sit bones. Slowly bring your feet, legs and upper back down towards the floor. If you suffer with any pain in your back, you can bend the legs. Go as low as you can, making sure you can feel your core and abs engaged and working once you get to your lowest point. Hold it there, squeezing all your muscles together for the time specified.

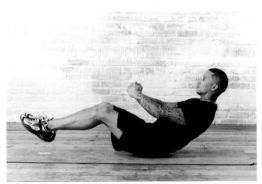

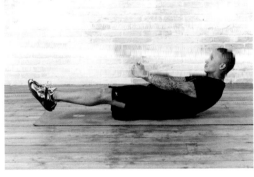

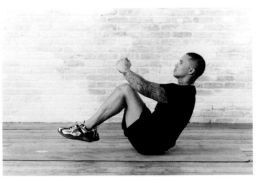

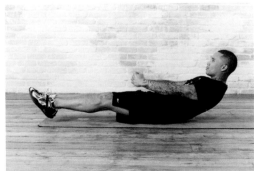

Alternating lunge jumps

1 With your legs in a split position, one leg in front of the other, keep both legs bent deep, with one knee down towards the floor.

2 Push up through both legs, jumping up as high as you can. As your feet leave the floor, start to swap the legs, with the front leg going backwards and the back leg coming forwards.

3 When your feet land back down to the floor, the opposite foot should be in front with the other foot behind. Smoothly bend the legs as you land and then jump back up, swapping in the legs over once again. Do this for the amount of reps required.

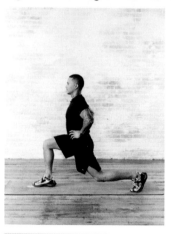 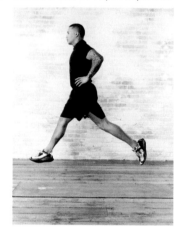 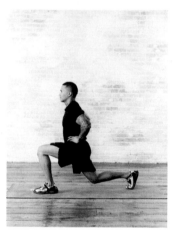

Reverse lunge knee drive jump

1 Step your leg back into a reverse lunge (page 37), bending at the knee.

2 Keep the front leg bent and stable, and as you come back up through the back leg, drive the knee up to the sky and jump up with your front leg straight. As the straight leg touches the floor step off the leg with the bent knee, back into reverse lunge and repeat for the amount of reps required. Change over to the other leg.

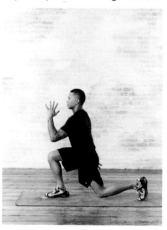 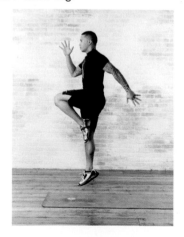

COOL-DOWN STRETCHES

Reverse prayer child's pose

Starting from a kneeling position, bring the palms of your hands together behind your back, fingers facing upwards. Lower your bum down towards your heels and fold forward, bringing your head down towards the floor. Bring your elbows back, pointing towards the ceiling.

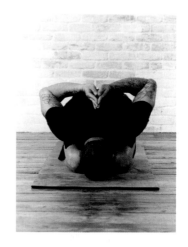

Gomukhasana eagle arms

Sit on the floor with one leg crossed over on top of the other, with your knees stacked on top of each other. Try to bring your knees and legs as tight around each other as possible, then bend your elbows and cross your forearms around each other so the palms of the hands are facing each other. Clamp the palms of the hands as flat together as possible.

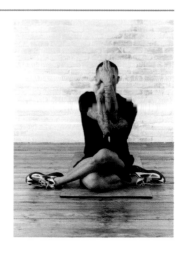

Seated spinal rotation

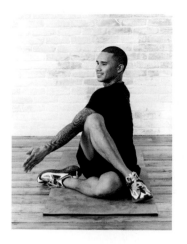

Sit with one leg on the floor and bending back towards your glutes. Bend the other knee and bring that foot to the outside of the opposite thigh. Starting with your arms out to the sides, bring the arm that corresponds to the flat leg across your body and straighten it over the outside of the upper leg, rotating your body through the spine. Straighten the opposite arm and reach behind you. Your upper body should be side on. Hold for the required time, then repeat on the other side. **Lying spinal rotation** – lie on your back and bring one knee up towards your chest and then across your body towards the floor, rotating through the spine. Bring the opposite arm flat across the floor, rotating through your torso.

Pigeon pose

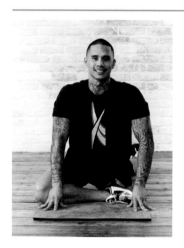

Start on all fours, hands shoulder width apart. Bring one knee forward in front of you, so it is just behind the wrist on that side. Bend the leg, allowing the knee to go out at a 45- or 90-degree angle, depending on your flexibility. Straighten the other leg out behind you, resting the knee on the floor. Either keep your hands on the floor with your arms straight or bring the elbows to the floor if you're more flexible. Repeat on the other side.

Child's pose

From a kneeling position, with the tops of the feet on the floor, bring your bum down towards your heels, keeping your arms straight out in front of you. Fold forward, place your hands flat on the floor, reaching forward, extending and stretching through the spine, and trying to bring your forehead down towards the floor.

Anjaneyasana

Kneel on the mat and bring one foot forward so the knee is bent. The back leg should be straight out behind you with the knee on the floor. Bring your thigh and hip flexor towards the floor resting on your knee and top of the foot. Open through your hips, pushing forwards, and open the chest. Extend your arms straight up, with hands together, or out to the sides.

CARDIOVASCULAR EXERCISE

Cardiovascular exercise is an important part of your training as it will contribute to your overall fitness: it increases your heart rate, works your muscles, strengthens your heart and increases your lung capacity. It helps to burn calories, and may help to prevent high blood pressure, diabetes and heart disease. It contributes to a healthier immune system and makes you feel good!

You are going to be doing three types of cardio exercise:

Aerobic
Running at a steady rate or beginning slowly and increasing the intensity.

Anaerobic
Short, explosive sprints.

Combination
Mixing aerobic and anaerobic when you're running but also during the workouts when you're using your own body weight.

I recommend doing cardiovascular exercise either in the morning before breakfast, or in the evening, but there are no hard and fast rules. It will normally take you up to 24 hours to recover fully from your cardio exercise. If a session has really taken its toll, take a bit longer to rest before you go again.

Cardio Workout #1

Any type of 'steady state' cardio exercise – e.g. running, cycling, swimming, rowing for a continous period of time, as stated.

Beginner: 15-20 minutes
Intermediate: 20-30 minutes
Advanced: 30-40 minutes

Cardio Workout #2

Explosive sprints at intervals using whichever exercise you prefer, e.g. running, rowing, skipping, cycling. Push as hard as you can for the required time, then rest for the required time, then repeat for the number of rounds stated.

Before beginning Cardio Workout #2, warm up for 5 minutes doing Cardio Workout #1.

Beginner
· Five rounds of: 45 seconds on, then 45 seconds off
· Rest for 1 minute
· Five rounds of: 30 seconds on, then 30 seconds off
· Rest for 1 minute
· Five rounds of: 15 seconds on, then 15 seconds off

Intermediate
· Five rounds of: 1 minute on, then 1 minute off
· Rest for 1 minute
· Five rounds of: 45 seconds on, then 45 seconds off
· Rest for 1 minute
· Five rounds of: 30 seconds on, then 30 seconds off

Advanced
· Ten rounds of 1 minute on, then 1 minute off
· Rest for 1 minute
· Ten rounds of: 30 seconds on, then 30 seconds off
· Rest for 1 minute
· Ten rounds of: 15 seconds on, then 15 seconds off

TESTING PHASE AND INITIATION

You must test yourself and gauge your level of fitness before launching into the 12-week programme. If you cannot do the Fitness Test, Flexibility Test and Strength Test here easily and perfectly, one after the other, start your training with the Initiation on this page. If you can do all three tests with ease, go straight into Beginner: Week 1 on page 68.

Record the results of the three tests so you can check back on them later and track your progress. If you did the Initiation, redo the Testing Phase after to see if you've improved and you're ready to start the programme.

Fitness test

1 ▶ Walking burpee chest to floor (*page 27*) – can you do more than 8 reps in one minute?

2 ▶ Running high knee (*page 40*) – can you go for 1 minute without feeling exhausted?

Flexibility test

1 ▶ Malasana stretch hold (*page 29*) – can you do/hold this pose?

2 ▶ Downward facing dog (*page 26*) – can you hold this pose for more than 30 seconds?

3 ▶ Start in downward dog and step one foot forwards between the hands (*page 26*), and then the other foot – is this easy to do?

Strength test

1 ▶ Press-up on knees (*page 24*) – can you do 10 reps?

2 ▶ Straight arm plank (*page 24*) – can you hold this for 20 seconds?

3 ▶ Squat (*page 23*) – can you do 10 reps going down to 90 degrees?

Initiation

If you have struggled to complete the 3 tests above with ease, start with this Initiation before the 12-week programme.

Do this initiation 3–4 times in a week. After the first week, do the Fitness Test, Flexibility Test and Strength Test again and see if you're ready to start the Beginner workout.

Dynamic stretch warm-ups
· Forward leg kick (*page 19*)
· Walking high knee (*page 20*)
· Walking heel to bum (*page 20*)
· Hip rotation (*page 20*)
· Forward and back arm circle (*page 21*)
· Floor wrist stretch (*page 22*)

Exercises
· Squat on sofa or low chair (*page 23*) – 3 sets of 10 reps and 30 seconds between each set
· Straight arm plank (*page 24*) – 10 seconds
· Walking burpee chest to floor (*page 27*) – 5 reps
· High level lunge (*page 24*) – hold for 20 seconds
· Leg raise (*page 34*) – 10 reps
· Elbow plank (*page 27*) – 20 seconds
· Press-up on knees (*page 24*) – 5 reps
· Utthita trikonasana (*page 193*) – 5 breaths each side
· Padangusthasana (*page 192*) – 5 breaths

BEGINNER – FULL BODY WORKOUT (WEEKS 1–4)

Optional 15 minutes' Cardio Workout #1 of your choice *(page 53)*, before or after the workout.

Dynamic stretch warm-ups, 1 minute each
· Forward leg kick *(page 19)*
· Walking high knee *(page 20)*
· Walking heel to bum *(page 20)*
· Hip rotation *(page 20)*
· Forward and back arm circle *(page 21)*
· Floor wrist stretch *(page 22)*

Exercises
Do 3 consecutive rounds of:
· Star jump *(page 23)* – 30 reps
· Walking high knee *(page 20)*– 30 reps
· Squat on sofa or low chair *(page 23)* – 10 reps
· High level lunge *(page 24)* – hold 10 seconds each side
· Straight arm plank *(page 24)* – 15 seconds
Rest 15 seconds

(For all the exercises here below, in weeks 3 & 4 increase everything by 2 reps except where reps are included in brackets.)

Do 2 consecutive rounds, 30 seconds' rest between each round, of:
· Press-up on knees *(page 24)* – 10 reps
· Plank press-up on knees *(page 25)* – 10 each side
· Walking mountain climber *(page 25)* – 20 reps
No rest between exercises

Do 2 consecutive rounds, 30 seconds' rest between each round, of:
· Straight arm plank step-out *(page 25)* – 20 reps
· Plank to downward facing dog *(page 26)* – 5 reps (weeks 3 & 4: 8 reps)
· Walking burpee chest to floor *(page 27)* – 5 reps (weeks 3 & 4: 8 reps)

· Elbow plank *(page 27)* – 15 seconds (weeks 3 & 4: 20 seconds)
· Slow glute kick pulse *(page 28)* – 20 reps each leg
· Slow donkey kick *(page 28)* – 20 reps each leg
· Reverse leg raise *(page 29)* – 20 reps

Do 2 consecutive rounds, 30 seconds' rest between each round, of:
· Sumo squat *(page 28)* – 10 reps
· Squat floor touches *(page 30)* – 15 reps (weeks 3 & 4: 18 reps)
· Static lunge *(page 28)* – 10 reps each leg
· Alternating side lunge *(page 38)* – 10 reps each side
· Squat hold on wall *(page 30)* – 20 seconds (weeks 3 & 4: 25 seconds)
No rest between exercises

Do 2 consecutive rounds, 20 seconds' rest between each round, of:
· Utthita trikonasana both sides *(page 193)* – 5 breaths each
· Utthita Parsvakonasana *(page 195)* – 5 breaths each side
· Padangusthasana *(page 192)* – 5 breaths
· Reverse prayer child's pose *(page 51)* – 5 breaths each side
· Leg raise and butt lift *(page 30)* – 10 reps
· Knee raise *(page 31)* – 10 reps
· Boat pose *(page 31)* – 10 seconds (weeks 3 & 4: 20 seconds)
No rest between exercises

Cool-down stretches, 5 breaths each (each side if required)
· Anjaneyasana *(page 52)*
· Lying spinal rotation *(page 52)*
· Pigeon pose *(page 52)*
· Child's pose *(page 52)*

BEGINNER – UPPER BODY WORKOUT (WEEKS 1–4)

Optional 15 minutes' Cardio Workout #1 of your choice *(page 53)*, before or after the workout.

Dynamic stretch warm-ups, 1 minute each
· Forward leg kick *(page 19)*
· Hip rotation *(page 20)*
· Forward and back arm circle *(page 21)*
· Lateral arm circle *(page 21)*
· Bear hug *(page 21)*
· Floor wrist stretch *(page 22)*

Exercises
Do 2 consecutive rounds of:
· Walking high knee *(page 20)* – 30 reps
· Jogging high knee *(page 31)* – 50 reps
· Straight arm walk-out *(page 32)* – 10 reps
· Straight arm plank *(page 24)* – 20 seconds

(For all the exercises here below, in weeks 3 & 4 increase everything by 5 reps except where reps are included in brackets.)

· Controlled negative full press-up *(page 32)* – 5 reps x 3 sets with 30 seconds' rest between each set
· Press-up on knees *(page 24)* – 10 reps x 3 sets with 30 seconds' rest between each set
· Tricep press-up on knees *(page 32)* – 5 reps x 3 sets with 30 seconds rest between each set

Do 2 consecutive rounds, 30 seconds' rest between each round, of:
· Downward facing dog, knee to tricep touch *(page 33)* – 10 reps each leg
· Corkscrew *(page 33)* – 10 reps each side (weeks 3 & 4: 14 reps)
· Elbow plank hip dip *(page 34)* – 16 reps (weeks 3 & 4: 20 reps)
· Elbow side plank *(page 34)* – 20 seconds

Do 2 consecutive rounds, 50 seconds' rest between each round, of:
· Single leg knee to chest *(page 35)* – 10 reps (weeks 3 & 4: 16 reps)
· Leg raise *(page 34)* – 10 reps
· Scissors *(page 35)* – 30 reps (weeks 3 & 4: 40 reps)
· Flutters *(page 36)* – 30 reps (weeks 3 & 4: 40 reps)
· Boat pose *(page 31)* – 20 seconds
· Back extension *(page 36)* – 20 reps
· Arch *(page 37)* – 20 seconds
No rest between exercises

Cool-down stretches, 5 breaths each (each side if required)
· Reverse prayer child's pose *(page 51)*
· Gomukhasana eagle arms *(page 51)*
· Anjaneyasana *(page 52)*
· Setu Bandhasana *(page 204)*

BEGINNER – LOWER BODY WORKOUT (WEEKS 1–4)

Optional 15 minutes' Cardio Workout #1 of your choice *(page 53)*, before or after the workout.

Dynamic stretch warm-ups, 1 minute each
· Forward leg kick *(page 19)*
· Lateral leg kick *(page 19)*
· Walking heel to bum *(page 20)*
· Hip rotation *(page 20)*
· Forward and back arm circle *(page 21)*

Exercises
Do 2 consecutive rounds of:
· Walking high knee *(page 20)* – 30 reps
· Star jump *(page 23)* – 50 reps
· Squat on sofa or low chair *(page 23)* – 10 reps
· High level lunge *(page 24)* – hold 10 seconds each side

· Malasana stretch hold *(page 29)* – 20–30 seconds
· Slow glute kick pulse *(page 28)* – 20 reps each leg
· Slow donkey kick *(page 28)* – 20 reps each leg
· Reverse leg raise *(page 29)* – 20 reps

(For all the exercises here below, in weeks 3 & 4 increase everything by 5 reps except where reps are included in brackets.)

Do 2 consecutive rounds, 1 minute's rest between each round, of:
· Squat on sofa or low chair *(page 23)* – 10 reps
· Sumo squat *(page 28)* – 10 reps
· Sumo squat *(page 28)* – hold at bottom 15 seconds
· Alternating forward lunges *(page 37)* – 10 reps

· Alternating reverse lunges *(page 37)* – 10 reps
· Static lunge *(page 28)* – 10 reps each leg
· Squat jump on sofa or low chair *(page 23)* – 10 reps
No rest between exercises

Do 3 consecutive rounds, 1 minute's rest between each round, of:
· Reverse lunge *(page 37)* – 15 reps each leg
· Side lunge *(page 38)* - 10 reps each leg
· Squat hold on wall *(page 30)* – 20 seconds
No rest between exercises

Do 3 consecutive rounds of:
· Crunch *(page 38)* – 20 reps
· Sit up *(page 38)* – 20 reps
· Reverse leg raise *(page 29)* – 20 reps
· Reverse plank *(page 38)* – 10 seconds
No rest between exercises

Cool-down stretches, 5 breaths each (each side if required
· Utthita trikonasana *(page 193)*
· Utthita parsvakonasana *(page 193)*
· Padangusthasana *(page 192)*
· Anjaneyasana *(page 52)*
· Pigeon pose *(page 52)*

INTERMEDIATE – FULL BODY WORKOUT (WEEKS 5–8)

Optional 20 minutes' Cardio Workout #1 of your choice (page 53), before or after the workout.

Dynamic stretch warm-ups, 1 minute each
· Forward leg kick (page 19)
· Walking high knee (page 20)
· Walking heel to bum (page 20)
· Hip rotation (page 20)
· Forward and back arm circle (page 21)
· Floor wrist stretch (page 22)

Exercises
Do 2–3 consecutive rounds of:
· Star jump (page 23) – 30 reps
· Jogging high knee (page 31) – 50 reps
· Squat (page 23) – 20 reps
· High level lunge pulse (page 39) – 15 reps each leg
· Straight arm plank (page 24) – 25 seconds

(For all the exercises here below, in weeks 7 & 8 increase everything by 2 reps except where reps are included in brackets.)

Do 3 consecutive rounds, 30 seconds' rest between each round, of:
· Full press-up (page 37) – 8 reps (weeks 7 & 8: 10–12 reps)
· Press-up on knees (page 24) – 10 reps
· Plank press-up (page 44) – 8 each side (weeks 7 & 8: 10 reps)
· Walking mountain climber (page 25) – 30 reps
No rest between exercises

· Shoulder tap (page 39) – 20 reps
· Snap jump (page 38) – 20 reps
· Plank to downward facing dog (page 26) – 10 reps
· Burpee chest to floor (page 40) – 10 reps
· Running high knee (page 40) – 20 seconds (weeks 7 & 8: 30 seconds)
Rest 20 seconds

Do 2 consecutive rounds, 30 seconds' rest between each round, of:
· Straight arm side plank, lift leg (page 42) – 15 seconds each leg (weeks 7 & 8: 30 seconds)
· Flip the dog (page 40) – hold 10 seconds, repeat both sides
· Elbow plank pike walk-in (page 41) – 5 reps (weeks 7 & 8: 8 reps)

Do 2 consecutive rounds, 30 seconds' rest between each round, of:)
· Low squat (page 41) – 10 reps
· Sumo squat (page 28) – 15 reps (weeks 7 & 8: 18 reps)
· Forward lunge (page 37) – 12 reps each side
· Squat holds (page 41) – hold at bottom 30 seconds (weeks 7 & 8: no change)
No rest between exercises

Do 2 consecutive rounds, 30 seconds' rest between each round, of:
· Leg raise (page 34) – 15 reps (weeks 7 & 8: no change)
· Knee raise (page 31) – 15 reps (weeks 7 & 8: no change)
· Boat pose (page 31) – 20 seconds (weeks 7 & 8: 25 seconds)
· Reverse plank (page 38) – 20 seconds (weeks 7 & 8: 25 seconds)
No rest between exercises

· Utthita trikonasana (page 193) – 5 breaths each side
· Utthita parsvakonasana (page 195) – 5 breaths
· Padangusthasana (page 192) – 5 breaths
· Reverse prayer child's pose (page 51) – 5 breaths each side

Cool-down stretches, 5 breaths each (each side if required)
· Anjaneyasana (page 52)
· Lying spinal rotation (page 52)
· Pigeon pose (page 52)

INTERMEDIATE – UPPER BODY WORKOUT (WEEKS 5–8)

Optional 20 minutes' Cardio Workout #1 of your choice (*page 53*), before or after the workout.

Dynamic stretch warm-ups, 1 minute each
· Forward leg kick (*page 19*)
· Hip rotation (*page 20*)
· Forward and back arm circle (*page 21*)
· Lateral arm circle (*page 21*)
· Bear hug (*page 21*)
· Floor wrist stretch (*page 22*)

Exercises
Do 2 consecutive rounds, 30 seconds' rest between each round, of:
· Walking high knee (*page 20*) – 30 reps
· Star jump (*page 23*) – 50 reps
· Straight arm walk-out with alternating knee drive jump (*page 42*) – 10 reps
· Straight arm plank (*page 24*) – 20 seconds

(For all the exercises here below, in weeks 7 & 8 increase everything by 5 reps or seconds except where reps or seconds are included in brackets.)

30 seconds' rest between each set of:
· Full press-up (*page 37*) – as many as you can until you can't do any more – then straight into press-up on knees (*page 24*) – 10 reps
· Tricep press-up on knees (*page 32*) – 10 reps x 3 sets
No rest between exercises

Do 2 consecutive rounds, 30 seconds' rest between each round, of:
· Plank press-up on knees (*page 25*) – 10 reps each side
· Downward facing dog, knee to tricep touch (*page 33*) – 15 reps each leg
· Elbow plank hip dip (*page 34*) – 10 reps (weeks 7 & 8: 16 reps)
· Side elbow plank hip dips (*page 43*) – 20 seconds each side

Do 2 consecutive rounds of:
· Flip the dog (*page 40*) – hold 15 seconds each side
· Elbow plank pike walk-in (*page 41*) – 8 reps (weeks 7 & 8: 10 reps)
No rest between exercises

Do 2 consecutive rounds, 30 seconds' rest between each round, of:
· Single leg knee to chest (*page 35*) – 16 reps (weeks 7 & 8: 20 reps)
· Leg raise (*page 34*) – 15 reps
· Scissors (*page 35*) – 50 reps (weeks 7 & 8: 60 reps)
· Flutters (*page 36*) – 50 reps (weeks 7 & 8: 60 reps)
· Boat pose (*page 31*) – 30 seconds
· Back extension (*page 36*) – 30 reps
· Arch (*page 37*) – 30 seconds
No rest between exercises

Cool-down stretches, 5 breaths each (each side if required)
· Reverse prayer child's pose (*page 51*)
· Gomukhasana eagle arms (*page 51*)
· Anjaneyasana (*page 52*)
· Setu Bandhasana (*page 204*)

INTERMEDIATE – LOWER BODY WORKOUT (WEEKS 5–8)

Optional 20 minutes' Cardio Workout #1 of your choice *(page 53)*, before or after the workout.

Dynamic stretch warm-ups, 1 minute each
· Forward leg kick *(page 19)*
· Lateral leg kick *(page 19)*
· Walking heel to bum *(page 20)*
· Hip rotation *(page 20)*
· Forward and back arm circle *(page 21)*

Exercises
Do 2 consecutive rounds of:
· Walking high knee *(page 20)* – 30 reps
· Star jump *(page 23)* – 50 reps
· Squat *(page 23)* – 15 reps
· Alternating forward lunges *(page 37)* – 20 reps
No rest between exercises

· Malasana stretch hold *(page 29)* – 45 seconds

(For all the exercises here below, in weeks 7 & 8 increase everything by 5 reps or seconds except where reps or seconds are included in brackets.)

Do 2 consecutive rounds, 1 minute's rest between each round, of:
· Squat *(page 23)* – 15 reps
· Sumo squat *(page 28)* – 10 reps straight into sumo squat – hold at bottom 15 seconds
· Squat jump *(page 43)* – 10 reps
· Alternating forward lunges *(page 37)* – 20 reps (weeks 7 & 8: 30 reps)
· Alternating reverse lunges *(page 37)* – 20 reps (weeks 7 & 8: 30 reps)
· Static lunge *(page 28)* – 12 reps each leg (weeks 7 & 8: 15 reps)

· Side lunge *(page 38)* – 12 reps each side (weeks 7 & 8: 15 reps)
No rest between exercises

Do 2 consecutive rounds, 1 minute's rest between each round, of:
· Reverse lunge knee drive jump *(page 50)* – 10 reps each leg
· Squat jump touchdown *(page 43)* – 20 reps
· Squat hold on wall *(page 30)* – 30 seconds
No rest between exercises

· Leg raise and butt lift *(page 30)* – 15 reps
· Sit up *(page 38)* – 20 reps
· Reverse leg raise *(page 29)* – 30 reps
· Reverse plank *(page 38)* – 30 seconds
· Utthita trikonasana *(page 193)* – 5 slow breaths each side

Cool-down stretches, 5 breaths each (each side if required)
· Utthita parsvakonasana *(page 195)*
· Padangusthasana *(page 192)*
· Anjaneyasana *(page 52)*
· Pigeon pose *(page 52)*

ADVANCED – FULL BODY WORKOUT (WEEKS 9–12)

As this is an advanced workout, the yoga sequences are incorporated into the exercises. Optional 30 minutes' Cardio Workout #1 of your choice (*page 53*), before or after the workout.

Dynamic stretch warm-ups, 1 minute each
· Forward leg kick (*page 19*)
· Lateral leg kick (*page 19*)
· Walking high knee (*page 20*)
· Walking heel to bum (*page 20*)
· Hip rotation (*page 20*)
· Forward and back arm circle (*page 21*)
· Floor wrist stretch (*page 22*)

Exercises
Do 3 consecutive rounds of:
· Star jump (*page 23*) – 30 reps
· Low squat (*page 41*) – 20 reps
· Running high knee (*page 40*) – 30 seconds
· Alternating forward lunges (*page 37*) – 20 reps
· One leg straight arm plank (*page 39*) –
  15 seconds each leg
Rest 20 seconds after the last round

(For all the exercises here below, in weeks 11 & 12 increase everything by 5 reps or seconds.)

· Full press-up (*page 37*) – 10 reps
· Controlled negative full press-up (*page 32*) –
  10 reps
· Plank press-up (*page 44*) – 10 each side
· One leg straight arm plank (*page 39*) –
  15 seconds each leg
· Walking mountain climber (*page 25*) – 30 reps
· Snap jump (*page 38*) – 30 reps
Rest 15 seconds

· One leg handstand jumps (*page 44*) – 10 reps
  each side
· Walking burpee chest to floor (*page 27*) –
  15 reps
· Lateral touchdown run (*page 44*) – 30 reps
· Elbow plank (*page 27*) – 30 seconds then walk
  feet in to elbow plank pike walk-in (*page 41*) and
  hold 10 seconds then walk feet back
Rest 15 seconds

Do 2 consecutive rounds of:
· Straight arm side plank, right hand down (*page 42*)
  – 15 seconds
· Flip the dog (*page 40*) – hold 15 seconds each side
· Full wheel (*page 45*) – 10 seconds
· Straight arm side plank, left hand down (*page 42*)
  – 15 seconds
· Flip the dog (*page 40*) – hold 15 seconds each side
· Full wheel (*page 45*) – 10 seconds
Rest 15 seconds after the last round

· Low squat (*page 41*) – 15 reps
· Sumo squat (*page 28*) – 15 reps
· Squat jump (*page 43*) – 15 reps

· One leg handstand jumps, right leg (*page 44*) –
  5 reps
· Step right leg forward into high level lunge
  (*page 24*) – hold 20 seconds
· Right leg forward static lunge (*page 28*) – 15 reps
· Right leg forward lunge (*page 37*) – 15 reps
· Right leg reverse lunge (*page 37*) – 15 reps
· Right leg forward Utthita trikonasana (*page 193*) –
  5 slow deep breaths
· Right leg forward Utthita parsvakonasana (*page
  195*) – 5 slow deep breaths
· Parsvottanasana, right leg forward (*page 197*) –
  5 slow deep breaths
Repeat whole round on the left side

Rest 20 seconds

Do 2 consecutive rounds of:
· Leg raise (*page 34*) – 20 reps
· Knee raise (*page 31*) – 20 reps
· V up (*page 45*) – 20 reps
· Boat pose (*page 31*) – 20 seconds
No rest between exercises

**Cool-down stretches, 5 breaths each
(each side if required)**
· Lying spinal rotation (*page 52*)
· Pigeon pose (*page 52*)
· Reverse prayer child's pose (*page 51*)

ADVANCED – UPPER BODY WORKOUT (WEEKS 9–12)

Optional 30 minutes' Cardio Workout #1 of your choice *(page 53)*, before or after the workout.

Dynamic stretch warm-ups, 1 minute each
· Forward leg kick *(page 19)*
· Hip rotation *(page 20)*
· Forward and back arm circle *(page 21)*
· Lateral arm circle *(page 21)*
· Bear hug *(page 21)*
· Floor wrist stretch *(page 22)*

Exercises
Do 2 consecutive rounds of:
· Jogging high knee *(page 31)* – 30 reps
· Star jump *(page 23)* – 50 reps
· Straight arm walk-out with alternating knee drive jump *(page 42)* – 16 reps
· Straight arm plank *(page 24)* – 30 seconds
· Straight arm plank rock *(page 45)* – 10 reps
Rest 30 seconds

(For all the exercises here below, in weeks 11 & 12 increase everything by 5 reps or seconds except where reps or seconds are included in brackets.)

50-second rest between each set of:
· Full press-up *(page 37)* – 15 reps
· Diamond press-up *(page 46)* – 5–10 reps x 3 sets

Do 2 consecutive rounds, 30 seconds' rest between each round, of:
· Tricep press-up and single arm raise *(page 47)* – 10 reps
· Plank press-up *(page 44)* – 5 reps each side
· Downward facing dog, knee to tricep touch *(page 33)* – 15 reps each leg
Rest 20 seconds

· One leg handstand jumps *(page 44)* (try to hold at the top for a few seconds, do against a wall each rep alternate the leg) – 10 reps
· Pincha single leg hold *(page 47)* (try to hold at the top for a few seconds, each rep alternate the legs) – 10 reps (weeks 11 & 12: 16 reps)

Do 2 consecutive rounds, 20 seconds' rest between each round, of:
· Straight arm side plank *(page 42)* – 30 seconds each side
· Flip the dog *(page 40)*– hold 15 seconds each side
· Full wheel *(page 45)* – 10 seconds
· Half press-up hold *(page 46)* – 10 seconds (weeks 11 & 12: 15 seconds)

Do 2 consecutive rounds, 20 seconds' rest between each round, of:
· V up *(page 45)* – 12 reps (weeks 7 & 8: 20 reps)
· Leg raise and butt lift *(page 30)* – 20 reps
· Boat pose scissors *(page 48)* – 30 reps (weeks 11 & 12: 50 reps)
· Boat pose flutters *(page 48)* – 30 reps (weeks 11 & 12: 50 reps)
· Boat pose pulses *(page 49)* – 30 reps (weeks 11 & 12: 50 reps)
· Boat pose *(page 31)* – 20 seconds
· Low boat pose *(page 49)* – 20 seconds
· Reverse plank *(page 38)* – 30 seconds
· Back extension *(page 36)* – 30 reps
· Arch *(page 37)* – 30 seconds

Cool-down stretches, 5 breaths each (each side if required)
· Reverse prayer child's pose *(page 51)*
· Gomukhasana eagle arms *(page 51)*
· Anjaneyasana *(page 52)*
· Setu Bandhasana *(page 204)*

ADVANCED – LOWER BODY WORKOUT (WEEKS 9–12)

Optional 30 minutes' Cardio Workout #1 of your choice *(page 53)*, before or after the workout.

Dynamic stretch warm-ups, 1 minute each
Forward leg kick *(page 19)*
Lateral leg kick *(page 21)*
Walking heel to bum *(page 20)*
Hip rotation *(page 20)*
Forward and back arm circle *(page 21)*

Exercises
Do 2 consecutive rounds of:
· Running high knee *(page 40)* – 30 reps
· Star jump *(page 23)* – 50 reps
· Low squat *(page 41)* – 20 reps
· Squat *(page 23)* – 20 reps
· Alternating forward lunges *(page 37)* – 20 reps
No rest between exercises

· Malasana stretch hold *(page 29)* – 30 seconds

(For all the exercises here below, in weeks 11 & 12 increase everything by 5 reps or seconds except where reps or seconds are included in brackets.)

Do 2 consecutive rounds, 1 minute's rest between each round, of:
· Low squat *(page 41)* – 15 reps
· Squat jump *(page 43)* – 10 reps
· Sumo squat *(page 28)* – 15 reps
· Sumo squat jump *(page 46)* – 10 reps
· Squat holds *(page 41)* – hold at bottom 20 seconds
· Forward lunge *(page 37)* – 20 reps each side (weeks 11 & 12: 30 reps each side)
· Reverse lunge *(page 37)* – 20 reps each side (weeks 11 & 12: 30 reps each side)

· Alternating lunge jumps *(page 50)* – 20 reps
· Side lunge *(page 38)* – 12 reps each side (weeks 11 & 12: 15 reps)

Do 2 consecutive rounds, 1 minute's rest between each round, of:
· Squat pulse *(page 48)* – 30 reps
· Reverse lunge knee drive jump *(page 50)* – 15 reps each leg
· Squat hold on wall *(page 30)* – 45 seconds (weeks 11 & 12: 1 minute)

Do 2 consecutive rounds, 30 seconds' rest between each round, of:
· V up *(page 45)* – 12 reps (weeks 11 & 12: 20 reps)
· Leg raise and butt lift *(page 30)* – 20 reps
· Boat pose scissors *(page 48)* – 30 reps (weeks 11 & 12: 50 reps)
· Boat pose flutters *(page 48)* – 30 reps (weeks 11 & 12: 50 reps)
· Boat pose pulses *(page 49)* – 30 reps (weeks 11 & 12: 50 reps)
· Boat pose *(page 31)* – 20 seconds
· Low boat pose *(page 49)* – 20 seconds
· Reverse plank *(page 38)* – 30 seconds
· Back extension *(page 36)* – 30 reps
· Arch *(page 37)* – 30 seconds

Cool-down stretches, 5 breaths each (each side if required)
· Utthita trikonasana *(page 193)*
· Utthita parsvakonasana *(page 195)*
· Padangusthasana *(page 192)*
· Anjaneyasana *(page 52)*
· Pigeon pose *(page 52)*

BETWEEN WORKOUTS

Work on your weaknesses

Working on your weaknesses is crucial in the process of becoming a better you. Improving the areas you're weaker in will allow you to become stronger and fitter all round, and therefore to perform better. We all love to work on the exercises we are good at because it makes us feel good about ourselves! But after a while of this, you'll feel frustration that there are some exercises or muscles that are letting you down. So you need to keep an eye on this and address it.

Outside of your 12-week programme, I want you to work on your weaknesses.

Of the exercises in the Testing Phase on page 54, is there anything you still struggle with, even if you've been following the programme for a few days now – an exercise or particular stretch?

If so, choose the exercise and do 3 sets of 10 reps with proper form. If it's a particular stretch, do 3 or 4 similar stretches (stretches or variations on the same stretch that tackle the same part of the body) and hold each one for about 3 minutes.

Do a re-energizing workout

If you're feeling a bit tired and need to reboot between regular workouts, I recommend this simple re-energizing workout.

Do 10-15 minutes of nice and easy jogging (outside, or indoors on the spot). Warm up slowly and gradually get faster until you reach 70% of your maximum effort.

Choose 1 upper body exercise from page 56, 1 lower body exercise from page 57 and 1 core exercise of your choice and do 3 sets of 15 reps.

Then finish off with this yoga stretching:
· 2 x Sun Salutation A *(page 188)*
· 2 x Sun Salutation B *(pages 189–191)*
· Utthita trikonasana *(page 193)* – 1 minute each side
· Padangusthasana *(page 192)* – 1 minute
· Paschimottanasana A *(page 199)* – 1 minute
· Baddha konasana *(page 202)* – 1 minute

Remember: don't over-reach

During your weeks of training – cardio or other workouts – if you start to feel consistently tired or unwell, if your moods change or your sleep is disrupted, you might need to take a few days off the workouts, as your body might be trying to tell you that it needs rest. Be sensitive to your body and its messages and listen to them. It's important to learn to understand your body and not to assume you're being lazy or defeatist if you need a bit of time off.

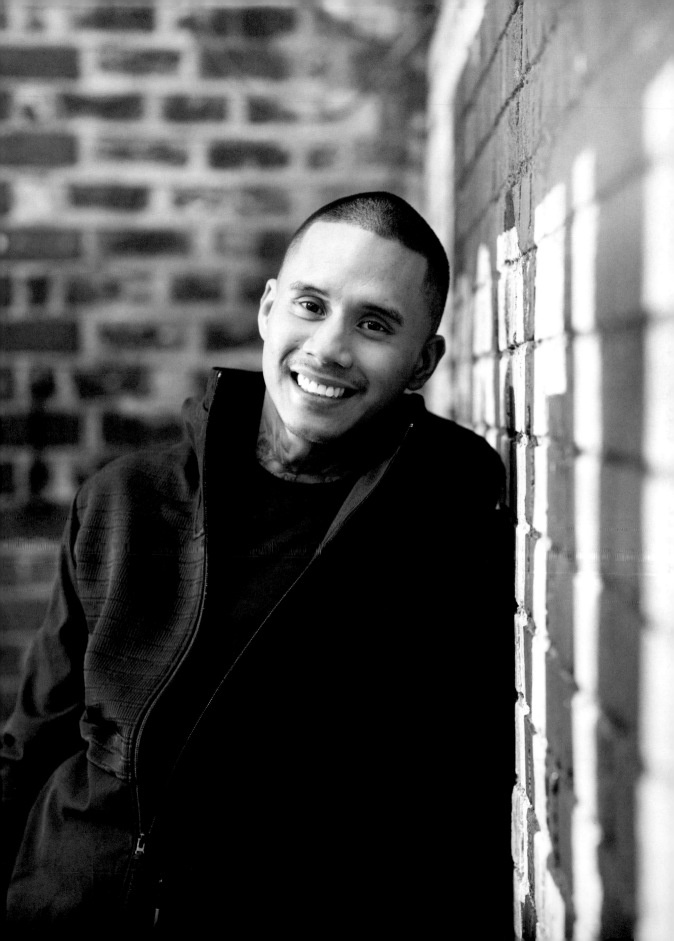

SUCCESS STORIES

Here are just a few 'before and afters' of some of my clients who did the 12-week programme and got amazing results.

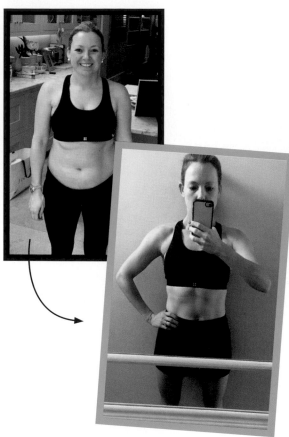

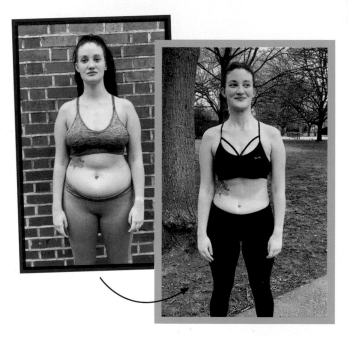

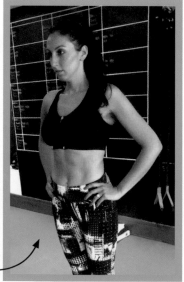

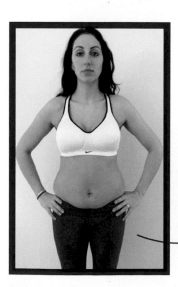

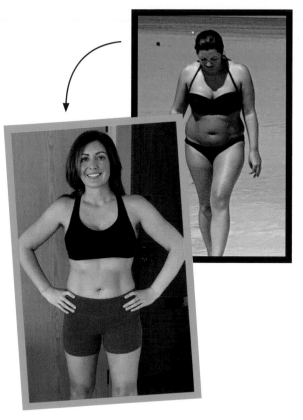
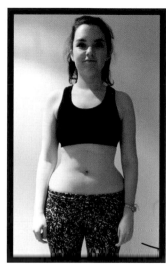
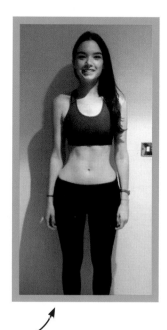
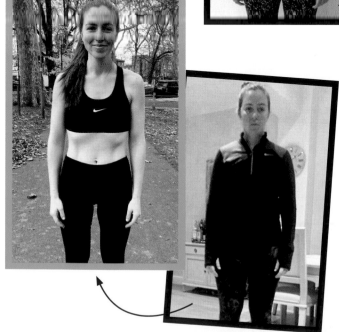

BEGINNER

			WEEK 1	WEEK 2
MONDAY	AM		Meditation: 4 minutes (page 211)	Meditation: 5 minutes (page 211)
	PM		Beginner – Full Body Workout (page 55)	Beginner – Full Body Workout (page 55)
TUESDAY	AM		Rest	Rest
	PM		Cardio Workout #2 (page 53)	Cardio Workout #2 (page 53)
WEDNESDAY	AM		Meditation: 4 minutes (page 211)	Meditation: 5 minutes (page 211)
	PM		Beginner – Upper Body Workout (page 56)	Beginner – Upper Body Workout (page 56)
THURSDAY	AM		Meditation: 4 minutes (page 211)	Meditation: 5 minutes (page 211)
	PM		The Yoga Practice: Beginner (page 186) + Work on your Weaknesses (page 64)	The Yoga Practice: Beginner (page 186) + Work on your Weaknesses (page 64)
FRIDAY	AM		Meditation: 4 minutes (page 211)	Meditation: 5 minutes (page 211)
	PM		Beginner – Lower Body Workout (page 57)	Beginner – Lower Body Workout (page 57)
SATURDAY	AM		Rest	Rest
	PM		Rest	Rest
SUNDAY	AM		Rest	Rest
	PM		Rest	Rest

		WEEK 3	**WEEK 4**
MONDAY	**AM**	Meditation: 5 minutes (page 211)	Meditation: 6 minutes (page 211)
	PM	Beginner – Full Body Workout (page 55)	Beginner – Full Body Workout (page 55)
TUESDAY	**AM**	Rest	Rest
	PM	Cardio Workout #2 (page 53)	Cardio Workout #2 (page 53)
WEDNESDAY	**AM**	Meditation: 5 minutes (page 211)	Meditation: 6 minutes (page 211)
	PM	Beginner – Upper Body Workout (page 56)	Beginner – Upper Body Workout (page 56)
THURSDAY	**AM**	Meditation: 5 minutes (page 211)	Meditation: 6 minutes (page 211)
	PM	The Yoga Practice: Beginner (page 186) + Work on your Weaknesses (page 64)	The Yoga Practice: Beginner (page 186) + Work on your Weaknesses (page 64)
FRIDAY	**AM**	Meditation: 5 minutes (page 211)	Meditation: 6 minutes (page 211)
	PM	Beginner – Lower Body Workout (page 57)	Beginner – Lower Body Workout (page 57)
SATURDAY	**AM**	Rest	Rest
	PM	Rest	Rest
SUNDAY	**AM**	Rest	Rest
	PM	Rest	Rest

INTERMEDIATE

		WEEK 5	WEEK 6
MONDAY	AM	Meditation: 7 minutes (page 211)	Meditation: 7 minutes (page 211)
	PM	Intermediate – Full Body Workout (page 58)	Intermediate – Full Body Workout (page 58)
TUESDAY	AM	Rest	Rest
	PM	Cardio Workout #2 (page 53)	Cardio Workout #2 (page 53)
WEDNESDAY	AM	Meditation: 7 minutes (page 211)	Meditation: 7 minutes (page 211)
	PM	Intermediate – Upper Body Workout (page 59)	Intermediate – Upper Body Workout (page 59)
THURSDAY	AM	Meditation: 7 minutes (page 211)	Meditation: 7 minutes (page 211)
	PM	The Yoga Practice: Intermediate (page 186) + Work on your Weaknesses (page 64)	The Yoga Practice: Intermediate (page 186) + Work on your Weaknesses (page 64)
FRIDAY	AM	Meditation: 7 minutes (page 211)	Meditation: 7 minutes (page 211)
	PM	Intermediate– Lower Body Workout (page 60)	Intermediate – Lower Body Workout (page 60)
SATURDAY	AM	The Yoga Practice: Intermediate (page 186) + Work on your Weaknesses (page 64)	The Yoga Practice: Intermediate (page 186) + Work on your Weaknesses (page 64)
	PM	Rest	Rest
SUNDAY	AM	Rest	Rest
	PM	Rest	Rest

		WEEK 7	WEEK 8
MONDAY	AM	Meditation: 8 minutes (page 211)	Meditation: 8 minutes (page 211)
	PM	Intermediate – Full Body Workout (page 58)	Intermediate – Full Body Workout (page 58)
TUESDAY	AM	Rest	Rest
	PM	Cardio Workout #2 (page 53)	Cardio Workout #2 (page 53)
WEDNESDAY	AM	Meditation: 8 minutes (page 211)	Meditation: 8 minutes (page 211)
	PM	Intermediate – Upper Body Workout (page 59)	Intermediate – Upper Body Workout (page 59)
THURSDAY	AM	Meditation: 8 minutes (page 211)	Meditation: 8 minutes (page 211)
	PM	The Yoga Practice: Intermediate (page 186) + Work on your Weaknesses (page 64)	The Yoga Practice: Intermediate (page 186) + Work on your Weaknesses (page 64)
FRIDAY	AM	Meditation: 8 minutes (page 211)	Meditation: 8 minutes (page 211)
	PM	Intermediate – Lower Body Workout (page 60)	Intermediate – Lower Body Workout (page 60)
SATURDAY	AM	The Yoga Practice: Intermediate (page 186) + Work on your Weaknesses (page 64)	The Yoga Practice: Intermediate (page 186) + Work on your Weaknesses (page 64)
	PM	Rest	Rest
SUNDAY	AM	Rest	Rest
	PM	Rest	Rest

ADVANCED

			WEEK 9	WEEK 10
MONDAY	AM		Meditation: 9 minutes (page 211)	Meditation: 9 minutes (page 211)
	PM		Advanced – Full Body Workout (page 61)	Advanced – Full Body Workout (page 61)
TUESDAY	AM		Rest	Rest
	PM		Cardio Workout #2 (page 53)	Cardio Workout #2 (page 53)
WEDNESDAY	AM		Meditation: 9 minutes (page 211)	Meditation: 9 minutes (page 211)
	PM		Advanced – Upper Body Workout (page 62)	Advanced – Upper Body Workout (page 62)
THURSDAY	AM		Meditation: 9 minutes (page 211)	Meditation: 9 minutes (page 211)
	PM		Cardio Workout #1 (page 53) + The Yoga Practice: Advanced (page 186)	Cardio Workout #1 (page 53) + The Yoga Practice: Advanced (page 186)
FRIDAY	AM		Meditation: 9 minutes (page 211)	Meditation: 9 minutes (page 211)
	PM		Advanced – Lower Body Workout (page 63)	Advanced – Lower Body Workout (page 63)
SATURDAY	AM		The Yoga Practice: Advanced (page 186) + Work on your Weaknesses (page 64)	The Yoga Practice: Advanced (page 186) + Work on your Weaknesses (page 64)
	PM		Rest	Rest
SUNDAY	AM		Rest	Rest
	PM		Rest	Rest

		WEEK 11	**WEEK 12**
MONDAY	AM	Meditation: 10 minutes (page 211)	Meditation: 10 minutes (page 211)
	PM	Advanced – Full Body Workout (page 61)	Advanced – Full Body Workout (page 61)
TUESDAY	AM	Rest	Rest
	PM	Cardio Workout #2 (page 53)	Cardio Workout #2 (page 53)
WEDNESDAY	AM	Meditation: 10 minutes (page 211)	Meditation: 10 minutes (page 211)
	PM	Advanced – Upper Body Workout (page 62)	Advanced – Upper Body Workout (page 62)
THURSDAY	AM	Meditation: 10 minutes (page 211)	Meditation: 10 minutes (page 211)
	PM	Cardio Workout #1 (page 53) + The Yoga Practice: Advanced (page 186)	Cardio Workout #1 (page 53) + The Yoga Practice: Advanced (page 186)
FRIDAY	AM	Meditation: 10 minutes (page 211)	Meditation: 10 minutes (page 211)
	PM	Advanced – Lower Body Workout (page 63)	Advanced – Lower Body Workout (page 63)
SATURDAY	AM	The Yoga Practice: Advanced (page 186) + Work on your Weaknesses (page 64)	The Yoga Practice: Advanced (page 186) + Work on your Weaknesses (page 64)
	PM	Rest	Rest
SUNDAY	AM	Rest	Rest
	PM	Rest	Rest

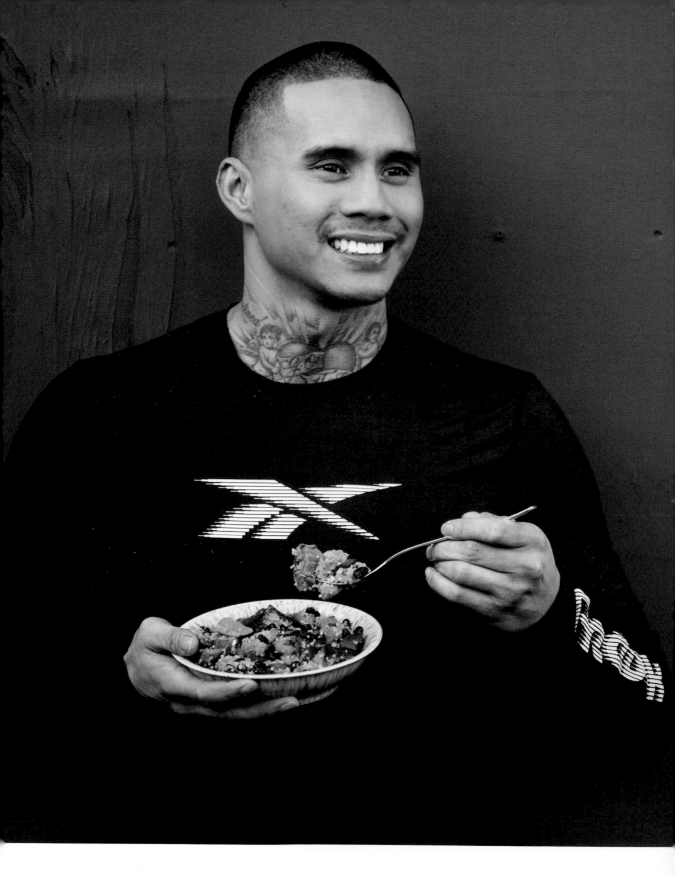

2

EAT THE FITTEST

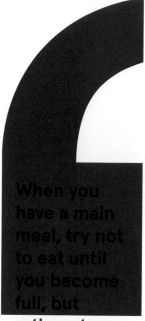

When you have a main meal, try not to eat until you become full, but **rather stop** when you're content. This will get easier the more you do it.

On the following pages you will find some of my favourite recipes – this is what I eat when I am training to give me energy. On pages 179–181 there are 3 sample weekly diet plans. You may find it easiest to follow these at first, and then as you become more confident in your food choices, adapt them so that they suit you.

Look at the suggestions on pages 78–79 and the recipes on pages 82–177 and make a shopping list. Aim to do a regular big shop to get the food that you like. Buy the best-quality ingredients that you can afford, and choose organic produce where possible.

Try to stick with this diet plan throughout the entire programme. I encourage you to be as creative as you want with your cooking, just stay within The Rules opposite.

You will be having three meals a day and one or two snacks. The meals you eat shouldn't be too large. Keep the portions of each type of food that make up the main meals to around the size of your fist. For vegetables, you can go up to a fist and a half, but for proteins stick to just a fist.

When you have a main meal, try not to eat until you become full, but rather stop when you're content. This will get easier the more you do it. The size of the meals should be enough so that you don't feel hungry, but should not leave you feeling full up.

As we are training, I want us to keep your carbohydrates to breakfast and lunch meals and really minimize them for any evening meals past 5–6pm. However if you feel your energy is really low, you can reload with a portion of carbs in an evening meal – but this has to be before 7pm!

Don't go hungry, eat accordingly when you need to, just keep it within the rules. Drink lots of water throughout the day to keep hydrated.

THE RULES

1 ▶ Try to minimize dairy – cut out cow's milk and use almond or coconut milk, for example, and also try to minimize your cheese intake. Cook using coconut oil or olive oil.

2 ▶ Aim for around 100g (3½oz) starchy carbs (such as pasta, rice or couscous) at breakfast and lunch. The rest of your carbs throughout the day should come from vegetables. If you are training twice a day and feeling low on energy, have some extra carbs with your evening meal.

3 ▶ Cut out white bread, white rice and white pasta and substitute them for the wholegrain or brown versions. Avoid processed foods.

4 ▶ If you are eating out in a restaurant, minimize the amount of alcohol you have, and try to order balanced meals with some carbs, protein and vegetables.

5 ▶ Try to stick to having your last meal of the day at around 7pm at the latest, unless you are training late. If you train first thing in the morning, just have lots of water and then eat after training; see also Rule 7. If you have training in the evenings, don't eat Meal 4 (your snack) too close to your session. Leave 3–4 hours with no food before training.

6 ▶ Don't go to bed feeling full up. Even feeling a tiny bit hungry is good. Having a chamomile tea with fresh mint will help you sleep and satisfy cravings if you have a sweet tooth in the evenings. See page 79 for other foods that might help you sleep.

7 ▶ If you lack energy before a workout, make one of the energy drinks (pages 82–83) an hour before your session.

8 ▶ Take your vitamins and probiotics and any other medications you may need. Seek medical advice from a doctor if you're unsure about any supplements you're taking.

9 ▶ Remember that the recipes are just examples of the types of foods to eat. If there's something that doesn't look good to you then change it, swap ingredients and make it your own.

10 ▶ Every 14 days of perfect eating you can have a cheat meal (any meal you are craving).

11 ▶ Drink lots of water and stay hydrated.

Recipe rules

▶ Use *either* the metric (grams, kilograms) measurements given in the recipes *or* the Imperial (ounces, pounds and cups) measurements in the brackets – do not switch between the two while you're making a recipe.

▶ The oven temperatures given in Celsius are for a conventional oven. If using a fan (convection) oven, lower the temperature by 10–20°C.

 = vegetarian

 = vegan

TY'S NUTRITION TIPS

Here are my tips to help you understand how to sustain a healthier diet and stay on track.

Storecupboard staples

These are the things that I stock up on – they are useful to have to hand for cooking, are long-lasting foods so are good to keep in the cupboards, make great snacks and can also help with reducing body fat.

1 ▶ Almond butter
A great food to have in the cupboard, you can eat with a piece of fruit or alone as a snack. Remember not to have too much: stick with 1 teaspoon per serving.

2 ▶ Coconut oil
This is great to cook with and to use for dressing your salads. It keeps you feeling full, which will help with cravings and keeping food portions controlled.

3 ▶ Chlorophyll liquid
This is available from health food stores. Add it to water as a drink. It has great benefits for the skin, aids with detoxification and helps with weight loss. Chlorophyll is found in fresh green plants so you can also add it to your diet by eating things like wheatgrass.

4 ▶ Brown rice
This is a long-lasting storecupboard staple and a healthier source of carbohydrate (which helps you to sustain energy levels for longer periods and decrease sugar cravings) than its white equivalent. Remember to stick to my portion rules (page 77).

5 ▶ Nuts (particularly almonds and walnuts)
These are a great source of proteins and omega-3 healthy fats. Can be stored for a long time. Only consume in small portions, such as a small handful.

6 ▶ Garlic
This is an essential ingredient for cooking – it adds flavour to foods, has proven health benefits and is low in calories. Just remember when eating garlic that it has a strong odour!

7 ▶ Oats
These are high in fibre and a fantastic source of carbohydrates which release over time. They have been proven in many studies to help lower cholesterol.

8 ▶ Quinoa
This is a wholegrain food packed with fibre, protein and minerals and is a great source of carbohydrates.

9 ▶ Extra virgin olive oil
This is a healthy fat which contains vitamin E. Use for dressing salads and cooking.

10 ▶ Seeds (particularly chia, hemp, ground flaxseed)
These are a great source of fibre – use for snacking or eating with breakfast meals. They will help to stave off hunger cravings.

11 ▶ Apple cider vinegar
Use for dressing salads, for generally adding flavour to dishes or as a condiment. Helps to reduce sugar spikes in the blood which helps with losing body fat.

12 ▶ **Green Tea**

This is a great drink to have between meals and has some health benefits – it's high in catechins which helps reduce visceral fat and cholesterol.

13 ▶ **Kidney beans**

These are a great source of carbohydrates and proteins in one. They contain amylase inhibitors that break down starches and other complex carbohydrates. They also prevent the release of simple sugars as well as delaying the digestion and absorption of carbohydrates.

14 ▶ **Ginger**

This is great for adding flavour to dishes. Add it to drinks and smoothies or use it in cooking. Ginger helps you to stay full for a longer period of time, which helps to reduce cravings and overeating. Ginger also aids digestion.

Food and drinks to help you sleep

Good-quality sleep is essential to overall health and will improve your energy levels during the day. If you are struggling to get to sleep or are experiencing post-dinner hunger pangs as you adjust to your new healthier diet, try including some of these foods.

Almonds

▶ A small handful of almonds is packed with protein and can completely satisfy my hunger. Besides staving off hunger, almonds are packed with nutrients that can improve sleep.

▶ Almonds (and some other nuts) contain melatonin, the body's natural sleep-regulating hormone.

▶ Almonds are packed with magnesium, an essential mineral which has been shown to reduce stress, stabilize our mood and promote better sleep quality.

Kiwi

▶ Often described as a superfood, kiwis are extremely nutritious and are low in calories. They contain high amounts of vitamins – one medium-sized fruit contains over 110% of your daily recommended vitamin C.

▶ Research shows that eating kiwi can have a beneficial effect on sleep – this is thought to be down to the fruit's high levels of antioxidants and serotonin.

Chamomile tea

▶ Chamomile is a traditional natural remedy for insomnia. Drinking chamomile tea before bed can help to relax the mind and body in preparation for a good night's sleep.

▶ Chamomile tea contains apigenin, an antioxidant which can help to promote good sleep quality.

▶ Studies have shown that people who drank chamomile tea every day for extended periods of time experienced improved, less interrupted sleep.

HOW TO CUT DOWN ON SUGAR

When adapting your diet to a healthier one, sugar may be the hardest thing to cut out. Many people experience strong sugar cravings, and there are different reasons why.

Below are some pointers to help you to think about ways you can change your habits, and also some clues to what might be behind your cravings.

I have also included my favourite alternatives to sugary snacks. Instead of giving in to your cravings, try one of my healthier options.

What time of day do you usually experience sugar cravings?

If you can predict the time that you are going to get cravings, it helps to have a healthier snack prepared, ready for that time. So if you regularly crave chocolate in the evenings, for instance, have a small slice of dark chocolate ready, but also a low-carb chocolate protein shake to help relieve your craving for the chocolate.

Are you eating enough nutrients throughout the day?

Often, people experience sugar cravings because they aren't getting enough of the right nutrients in their daily intake of foods. Perhaps think about consciously including more fibre, protein and good fats into your diet – this should have a positive effect on your cravings.

Are you getting enough sleep?

Sleep affects the hormones in your body which can contribute to how much your body craves certain foods, especially those that are high in calories or sweet. How much sleep are you getting? Try and relax a few hours before you sleep and do nothing too energetic before bed. See page 79 for some suggested foods to eat to improve sleep quality.

Are you hydrating enough and getting enough minerals into your diet?

Lacking in hydration can cause your body to crave sugar and high-calorie foods. Lacking in minerals and vitamins in your diet can also contribute to cravings. Make sure that you're staying hydrated throughout the day by drinking water, especially if you have worked out. Eat some fruit in the mornings, and make sure you eat correctly throughout the day – this should reduce your cravings. You can also supplement your diet by taking daily multivitamins.

Alternatives to try when craving sugar:

1 ▶ Swap your usual chocolate for a small amount of very dark chocolate

2 ▶ Drink a herbal tea with a touch of honey or maple syrup at night

3 ▶ Eat low-glycaemic index (GI) fruit (see below). Try and stick to these in the morning and afternoon when you need snack

4 ▶ A yogurt with a teaspoon of chia seeds stirred in

5 ▶ One or two dates or prunes

6 ▶ Smoothies (pages 83)

7 ▶ Small handful of nuts and some raisins

8 ▶ Low-calorie popcorn

Low-GI fruits:

▶ Cherries
▶ Plums
▶ Grapefruit
▶ Peaches (including canned – look for those in natural juices)
▶ Apples
▶ Pears
▶ Dried apricots
▶ Grapes
▶ Coconut
▶ Kiwi
▶ Oranges
▶ Strawberries

JUICES

These juices will keep for up to three days in a sealed glass bottle.

THE GREEN ONE

Packed with vitamins, this will help to support your immunity and reduce inflammation. It's ideal before a morning workout – energizing but not overly filling.

Makes about 500ml (2 cups)/serves 1

1 celery stick
⅛ fennel bulb
2.5cm (1in) piece of cucumber
½ kiwi, peeled or unpeeled as preferred
20g (½ cup) spinach leaves
½ Granny Smith apple, cored
3 ice cubes

Blend the ingredients together and serve.

THE RED ONE

Beetroot and ginger are great for your digestion. This is another juice that's good before a workout as it won't fill you up too much.

Makes about 500ml (2 cups)/serves 1

1 beetroot (beet), peeled and quartered
½ red apple, cored
5g (¼oz) fresh ginger, peeled
3 ice cubes

Add all the ingredients to a blender and top up with enough water to cover the ingredients. Blend and serve.

THE ORANGE ONE

If your energy is down and you think you might be coming down with something, make this and give your immune system a boost.

Makes about 500ml (2 cups)/serves 1

1 carrot, topped and tailed
5g (¼oz) fresh ginger, peeled
5g (¼oz) fresh turmeric, peeled
1 red apple, cored
3 ice cubes

Blend the ingredients together and serve.

SMOOTHIES

These smoothies will keep for up to three days in a sealed glass bottle.

THE VITAMIN ONE

I like to have this mega-nutritious smoothie on Monday when I have a hectic week ahead.

Makes about 500ml (2 cups)/serves 1

handful of spinach leaves
handful of kale leaves
¼ avocado
small slice of fresh ginger
juice of ½ lemon
1 red or green apple
400ml (1¾ cups) coconut milk or other
  dairy-free milk
1 tsp maple syrup

Blend the ingredients together and serve.

THE ENERGY ONE

This is good for boosting energy levels and makes a good snack if you're craving something sweet.

Makes about 500ml (2 cups)/serves 1

2 ice cubes
small handful of mango pieces
small handful of pineapple pieces
1 level scoop of vanilla protein powder,
  vegan if necessary
squeeze of fresh lime

Add all the ingredients to a blender and top up with enough water to cover the ingredients. Blend and serve.

THE POST-WORKOUT ONE

Drink this after a tough workout to feed the muscles and rejuvenate you.

Makes about 500ml (2 cups)/serves 1

2 ice cubes
½ banana
1 date
1 level scoop of chocolate protein powder,
  vegan if necessary

Add all the ingredients to a blender and top up with enough water to cover the ingredients. Blend and serve.

THE ON-THE-GO ONE

I take this with me to get me through the day without snacking and help see me through to the next meal.

Makes about 500ml (2 cups)/serves 1

2 ice cubes
handful of mixed berries
1 tbsp almond butter
1 level scoop of chocolate protein powder,
  vegan if necessary

Add all the ingredients to a blender and top up with enough water to cover the ingredients. Blend and serve.

BREAKFAST

V
BIRCHER MUESLI

You can prep this the night before, saving yourself time if you have a busy morning ahead. If you do soak this overnight, substitute the yogurt for almond milk and why not add a scoop of your favourite protein powder. It's a sustaining breakfast that's not too heavy.

Serves 1

1 apple
50g (½ cup) rolled oats
150g (⅔ cup) Greek yogurt
1 tbsp raisins

Grate the apple into a bowl, discarding the core and pips.

Add the remaining ingredients and mix everything together before serving.

Vg
PORRIDGE WITH BERRIES

This is my go-to winter warmer when I'm low on energy – lots of slow-release energy from those oats.

Serves 1

100ml (generous ⅓ cup) coconut milk
60g (½ cup) porridge oats
handful of mixed berries (blueberries, raspberries and strawberries)
1 tsp almond butter
1 tsp chia seeds
1 tsp hemp seeds

Warm the coconut milk in a pan over a medium heat for a few minutes. Add the porridge oats and stir as they warm through and start to thicken.

Once the oats have cooked and thickened transfer to a serving bowl.

Sprinkle the berries over the top of porridge. Add the almond butter in the middle and then sprinkle the chia and hemp seeds on top. Serve warm.

Vg

GRANOLA WITH FRUIT & SEEDS

V

COCONUT YOGURT BOWL

A classic breakfast but with added energy and protein from the seeds and berries. Goji berries have been eaten for thousands of years in their native Asia for their energy and numerous health benefits.

This couldn't be quicker to throw together. It's healthy, light and does the job. It also works as a mid-afternoon snack after a workout.

Serves 1

100g (½ cup) coconut yogurt
handful of blueberries (or strawberries or whatever berries prefer)
1 kiwi, peeled and sliced
honey, to taste (optional)

Serves 1

50g (1¾oz) organic, low-sugar granola
2 strawberries, sliced
handful of blueberries
1 tsp goji berries
1 tsp chia seeds
1 tsp hemp seeds
100ml (generous ⅓ cup) almond or coconut milk

Put the granola into a serving bowl.

Add the strawberries, blueberries and goji berries, then sprinkle over the chia and hemp seeds.

Pour over the almond or coconut milk to serve.

Place the coconut yogurt in a bowl, then sprinkle over the blueberries and kiwi slices. Serve with a small amount of honey If needed.

TY'S KILLER AVOCADO TOAST WITH MOJO VERDE & POACHED EGG

Are you craving something substantial and nutritious for breakfast? Here's your answer. Packed with nutrients and balanced by the carbs in the sourdough toast, it's good for a big day ahead.

Preheat your grill to a medium heat.

Grill the avocado, flat-side up, for 2–3 minutes.

Make the Mojo Verde. Mix the coriander (cilantro) and chilli together in a bowl. Squeeze over the juice from the lime. Add a small amount of honey if you prefer the taste to be less sharp. Add a teaspoon of the olive oil, season with salt and mix well. Set aside.

Poach the egg. Fill a medium pan with water and bring to the boil. Add the vinegar, turn the heat down to a rolling boil and crack the egg in, giving the water a slight stir.

Take the avocado out of the grill and toast both sides of the sourdough bread under the grill.

Once the bread is toasted, place it on a plate and smash the avocado onto your toast with a fork.

Remove the egg from the pan after 3–4 minutes using a slotted spoon and place on top of the avocado. Drizzle the Mojo Verde on top and serve.

Serves 1

½ avocado, peeled and stoned
1 bunch of coriander (cilantro), finely chopped
½ green chilli, finely chopped
1 lime
honey, to taste (optional)
1–2 tbsp olive oil
1 egg
1 tbsp white wine vinegar
1 slice of sourdough bread
sea salt

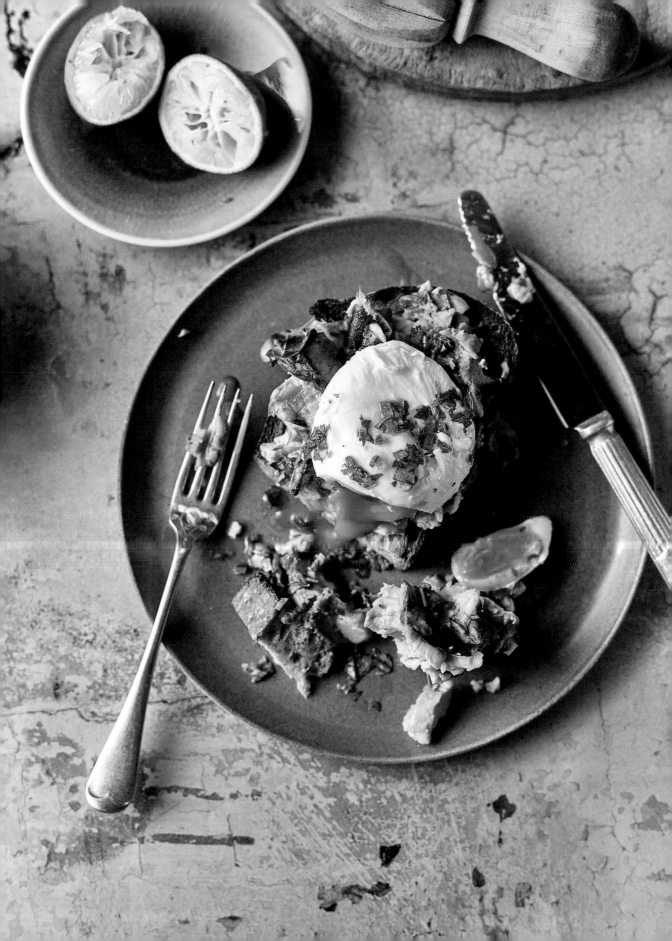

THE BEST BREAKFAST OMELETTE

This is one of my favourites when I want something hot, easy to make, lean and satisfying. There's protein from the egg whites and lots of nutrients in the egg yolks, plus iron in the spinach.

Beat the eggs together in a small bowl and season with salt and pepper.

Add the coconut oil to a frying pan over a medium heat. Once the pan is hot and the coconut oil has melted, add the onion and cook until soft and slightly browned. Add the cherry tomatoes and cook for 1½ minutes, then add the spinach and cook for a further 45 seconds or until soft but not overcooked.

Add the beaten eggs to the pan and swirl it around until the base of the pan is covered. Lower the heat and cook for a few minutes. Once the underside of the omelette is cooked and the top is solidifying, fold in half by flipping one half of omelette over the other. Cook for a couple more minutes, flip over and cook for another 30–60 seconds. Serve.

Serves 1

2 eggs
1 tbsp coconut oil
½ red onion, finely chopped
3 cherry tomatoes, halved
¼ red or green (bell) pepper
handful of baby spinach leaves
sea salt and freshly ground pepper

SCRAMBLED EGGS WITH SMOKED SALMON

Start the weekend right with this breakfast or brunch. It'll make you feel good for the rest of the day.

Beat the eggs with the egg white in a small bowl and season with salt and pepper.

Add the coconut oil to a pan over a medium heat. Once the pan is hot and the coconut oil has melted, add the spinach and/or kale to the pan, then the beaten eggs. Once around half of the egg has begun to solidify, add the smoked salmon and lower the heat.

Continue to cook, stirring, until the eggs have cooked through. Meanwhile, toast the slice of wholegrain bread.

Serve the eggs and salmon on top of the bread with some pepper. Garnish with dill.

Serves 1

2 eggs plus 1 egg white
1 tbsp coconut oil
handful of baby spinach (and/or kale) leaves
50g (1¾oz) smoked salmon, chopped
1 slice of wholegrain bread
sea salt and freshly ground pepper
fresh dill, torn, to garnish

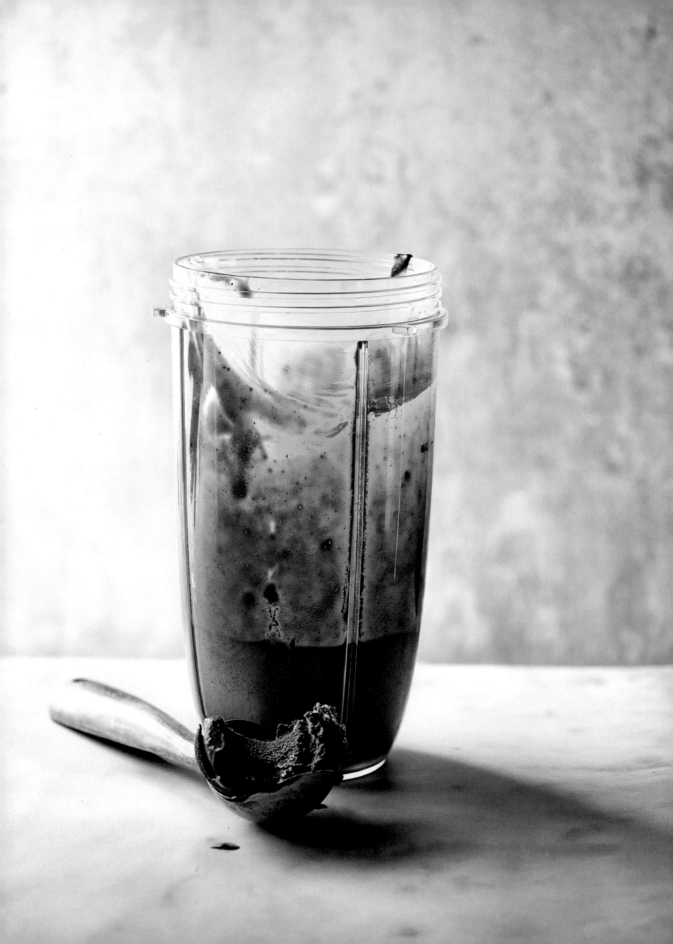

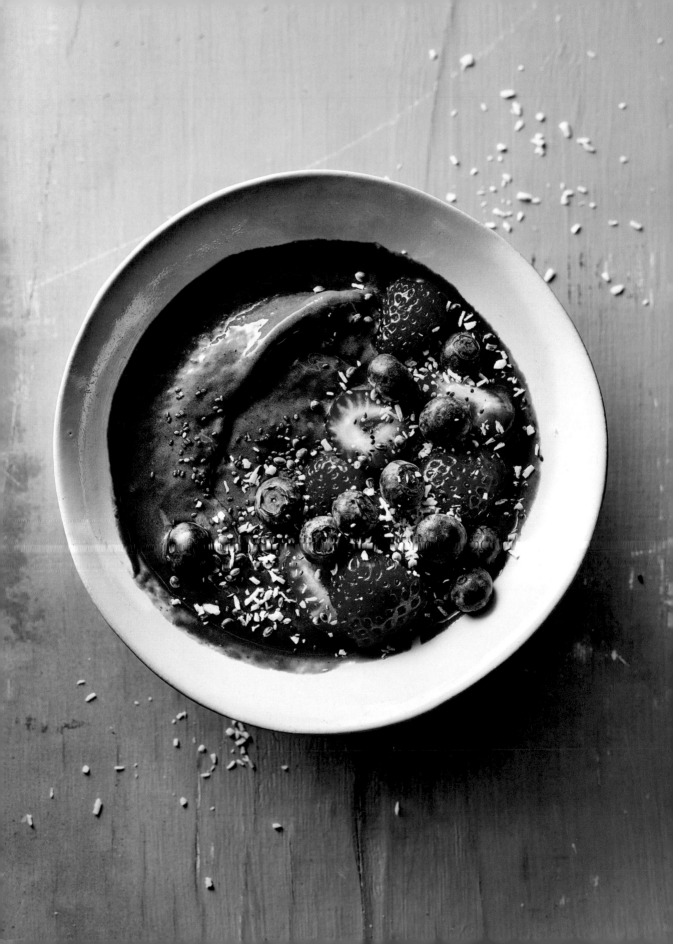

POST-WORKOUT ACAI BOWL

Vg

If your workout's really taken it out of you, you need a bowl of this. It's super easy to make and filled with fibre and protein. The hemp and chia seeds are great veggie sources of omega-3 fatty acids.

Add the açaí and banana to a blender and whizz together with the protein powder until combined.

Transfer to a bowl and add the strawberries and blueberries, then sprinkle over the seeds and coconut before serving.

Serves 1

100g (3½oz) frozen açaí purée
1 small–medium frozen banana
1 level scoop of protein powder,
  vegan if necessary
2–3 strawberries
handful of blueberries
1 tsp hemp seeds
1 tsp chia seeds
1 tsp desiccated coconut

MIGHTY GREENS ON SOURDOUGH TOAST

HEALTHY VEGGIE ENGLISH BREAKFAST

A lovely vegan or dairy-free option with good fats and carbs. You won't feel bloated after this.

Serves 1

½ avocado, peeled, stoned and roughly
  chopped
½ handful of baby spinach leaves
½ handful of kale, torn
1 tbsp balsamic vinegar
handful of cherry tomatoes, quartered
1 slice of sourdough bread
sea salt and freshly ground black pepper

Place the avocado in a bowl, mash with a fork, then add the spinach and kale and mix everything together. Add the balsamic vinegar and the tomatoes and mix again.

Toast the sourdough bread, then place on a plate. Spread the avocado mixture over the toast, season with salt and pepper and serve.

Opt for this on a Saturday or Sunday morning when you feel you deserve a treat. It's a healthier version of a Full English.

Serves 1

1 tbsp coconut oil
handful of Paris brown mushrooms,
  left whole
1 tomato, halved
1 egg
1 tbsp white wine vinegar
200g (7oz) baked beans
1 slice of sourdough bread

Bring a medium pan of water to the boil.

Meanwhile, heat the coconut oil in a frying pan over a medium–high heat. Add the mushrooms and cook for 2 minutes, then add the tomato halves, cut-side down, and cook for another couple of minutes.

Poach the egg. Fill a medium pan with water and bring to the boil. Add the vinegar, turn the heat down to a rolling boil and crack the egg in, giving the water a slight stir.

Stir the mushrooms and turn the tomato halves over. Heat the baked beans in a separate pan and toast the slice of bread.

Remove the egg from the pan after 3–4 minutes using a slotted spoon and put it onto a plate. Add the mushrooms, tomato and baked beans and serve with the warm toast.

SMOKED SALMON & CHILLI AVOCADO WITH POACHED EGG ON TOAST

Got a big day ahead and need a bigger breakfast? This is it! High in protein and good fats and made heartier with the egg and avocado. This'll get you going for a high-performance workout.

Poach the egg. Fill a medium pan with water and bring to the boil. Add the vinegar, turn the heat down to a rolling boil and crack the egg in, giving the water a slight stir.

Put the smoked salmon onto a plate, add the chopped avocado and then sprinkle over the chilli and season with salt and pepper.

Remove the egg from the pan after 3–4 minutes using a slotted spoon and place it on the toasted wholegrain or sourdough bread next to the avocado and salmon. Season with pepper and serve.

Serves 1

1 egg
1 tbsp white wine vinegar
40g (1½oz) smoked salmon
¼ avocado, peeled, stoned and chopped
1 red chilli, finely chopped
1 slice of wholegrain or sourdough bread, toasted
sea salt and freshly ground black pepper

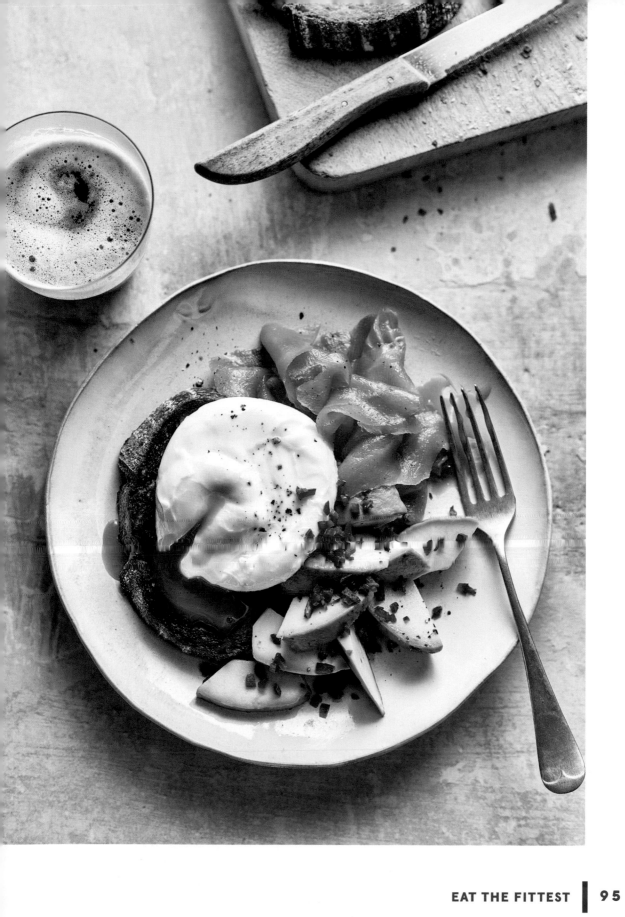

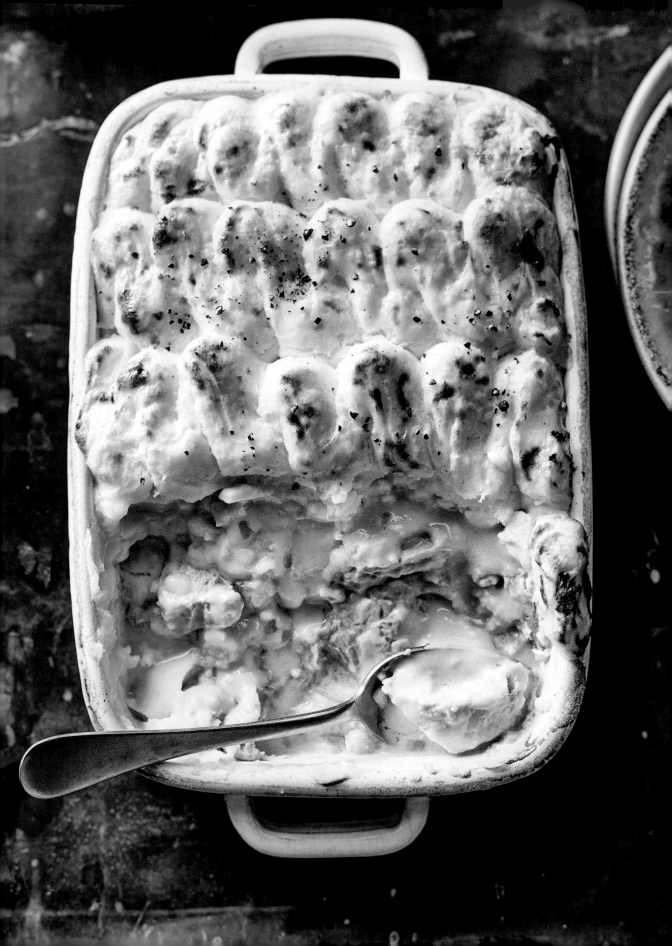

FIT FISH PIE WITH BROCCOLI & MANGETOUT

When you want to treat yourself to comfort food but keep on track at the same time, try this fit fish pie. Fish, especially oily fish, is a really good source of omega-3s.

Preheat the oven to 190°C/375°F/gas mark 5.

Place the potatoes in a large saucepan, add enough water to cover and a pinch of salt. Bring to the boil, then simmer for about 20 minutes or until soft.

Meanwhile, heat the butter in a frying pan and add the onion. Gently cook over a medium heat. Once the onion has softened, about 10–15 minutes, add the flour. Stir to combine and season with salt and pepper. Add the stock to the pan and heat, stirring, until you have a thick glossy sauce.

Place the fish into a pie dish, then pour over the sauce.

Once the potatoes are cooked, drain them and mash with a potato masher. Add the almond milk to ensure it is nice and smooth. Season with salt and pepper.

Transfer the mash to a piping bag and spread it out evenly on top of the fish mixture.

Place the pie in the oven and bake for 20–25 minutes or until golden on top.

While the pie is cooking, steam the broccoli and mangetout in a saucepan or in a microwave until just tender.

Remove the pie from the oven and serve alongside the broccoli and mangetout.

Serves 2

4 large potatoes, peeled and quartered
20g (1½ tbsp) butter
½ onion, finely chopped
20g (generous 2 tbsp) plain (all-purpose) flour
100ml (generous ⅓ cup) vegetable stock
200g (7oz) ready-prepared fresh fish pie mix
  or fish fillets of your choice
100ml (generous ⅓ cup) almond milk
200g (7oz) Tenderstem broccoli
200g (7oz) mangetout
sea salt and freshly ground black pepper

CRUNCHY COUSCOUS SALAD WITH WALNUTS & RAISINS

Vg

Summery, refreshing and light, this is ideal to make ahead and take with you in a container for a working lunch. Add the avocado at the last minute if you don't want it to go mushy.

Add 350ml (1½ cups) water to a saucepan and bring to the boil. Remove from the heat and add the couscous to the water with the raisins. Add the olive oil and season with a touch of salt. Cover and allow to rest for about 10 minutes until the couscous has absorbed all the water.

Using a fork, fluff up the couscous, separating all the grains.

Add the tomatoes, walnuts, cucumber, avocado and spinach and kale. Mix together thoroughly, add a squeeze of lemon juice and season with pepper.

Transfer to a bowl and serve.

Serves 2

150g (1 cup) couscous
2 tbsp raisins
1 tsp olive oil
6 cherry tomatoes, quartered
handful of walnuts, chopped
½ cucumber, diced
½ avocado, diced
handful of spinach and kale mix, chopped
1 lemon
sea salt and freshly ground black pepper

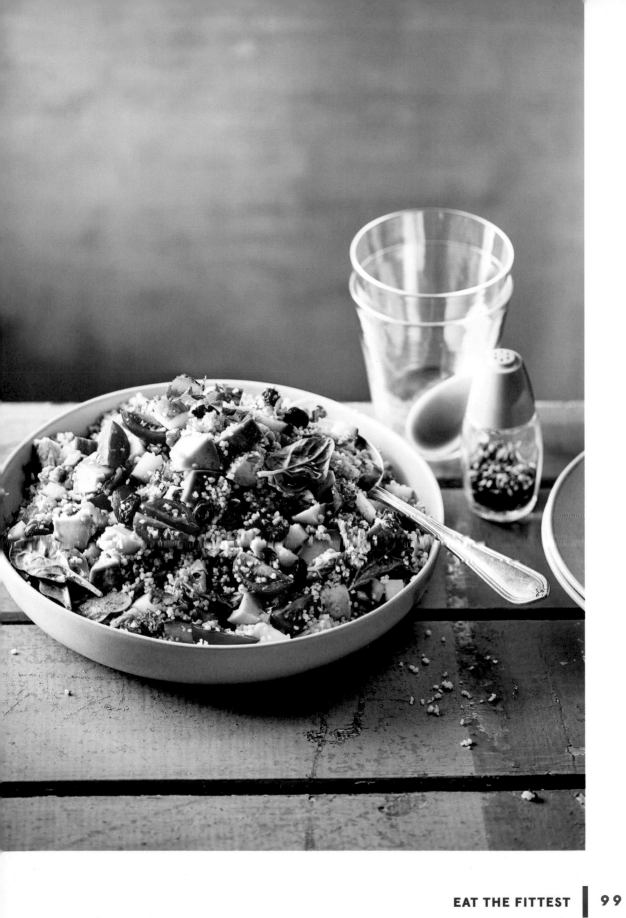

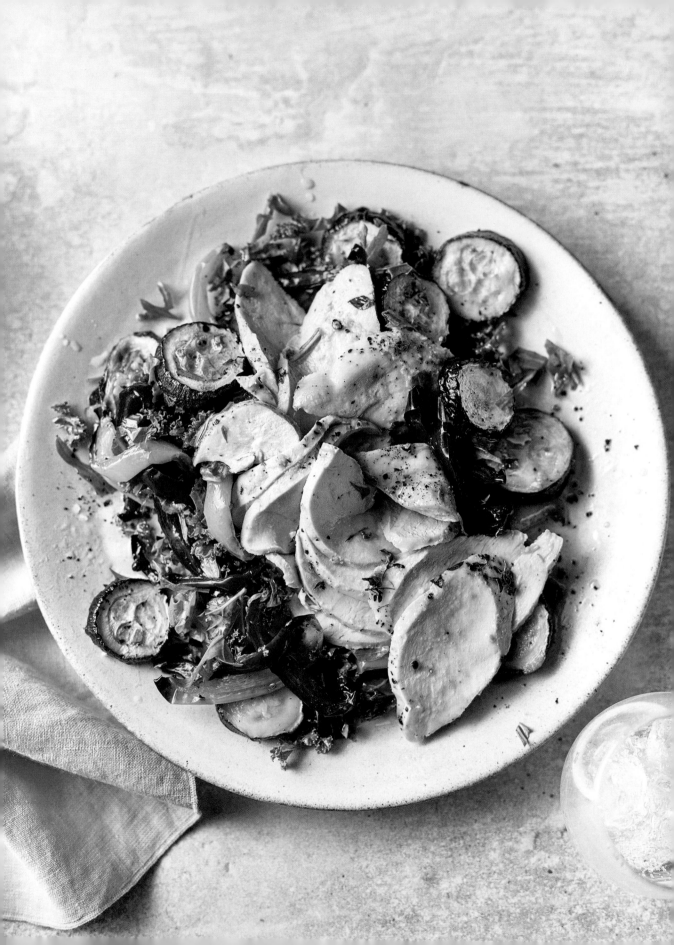

ROAST CHICKEN, PEPPER & COURGETTE SALAD

Because of the way the chicken, all the vegetables, thyme and garlic are cooked together, the flavours mingle and make a super flavoursome plate of food that's high in protein and still light and scrumptious.

Preheat the oven to 180°C/350°F/gas mark 4.

Place the chicken breast on a baking tray with the (bell) peppers and courgette (zucchini).

Put the garlic and thyme on top of the chicken breast and season with salt and pepper. Drizzle the chicken and vegetables with extra virgin olive oil. Put into the oven and bake for 25 minutes.

Put the finely sliced rocket (arugula) and kale into a large bowl.

Once the chicken is cooked, remove from the oven, lift the chicken onto a board and slice. Discard the thyme. Remove the courgette and peppers from the baking tray, leaving as much of the juices behind in the tray as possible. Put the cooked vegetables on top of the rocket and kale in the bowl, then lay the sliced chicken on top.

Squeeze the lemon into the baking tray with the cooking juices. Add a splash of extra virgin olive oil and stir. Season with salt and pepper and drizzle the dressing over the salad before serving.

Serves 1

1 chicken breast
½ red (bell) pepper, julienned
½ yellow (bell) pepper, julienned
1 small courgette (zucchini), sliced
1 garlic clove, crushed
2 thyme sprigs
handful of rocket (arugula), finely sliced
handful of kale, finely sliced
½ lemon
extra virgin olive oil
sea salt and freshly ground black pepper

THE KING OF SALADS, WITH GARLIC KING PRAWNS

After a tough morning workout, make this in a flash, take it outside and imagine you're on holiday. It's important to make time for yourself and not view cooking healthily as a chore – enjoy it!

Add the olive oil to a frying pan and fry the garlic with the chilli for 1 minute. Add the prawns (shrimp) and continue cooking for a few more minutes until the prawns are pink and opaque. Remove from the heat and set aside.

Put the spinach into a bowl, then add the avocado and tomatoes. Add the prawns and any juices from the pan, then sprinkle over the capers.

Add the dressing ingredients to a small bowl, adding more or less of each ingredient according to personal taste, and season with salt and pepper. Whisk the dressing, pour over the salad and toss before serving.

Serves 1

1 tbsp olive oil
3 garlic cloves, crushed
1 chilli, deseeded
150g (5¼oz) king prawns (shrimp)
2–3 handfuls of baby spinach
1 avocado, sliced
8 cherry tomatoes, halved
handful of capers

For the dressing
1 tbsp olive oil
1 tsp balsamic vinegar
½ tsp Dijon mustard
salt and freshly ground black pepper

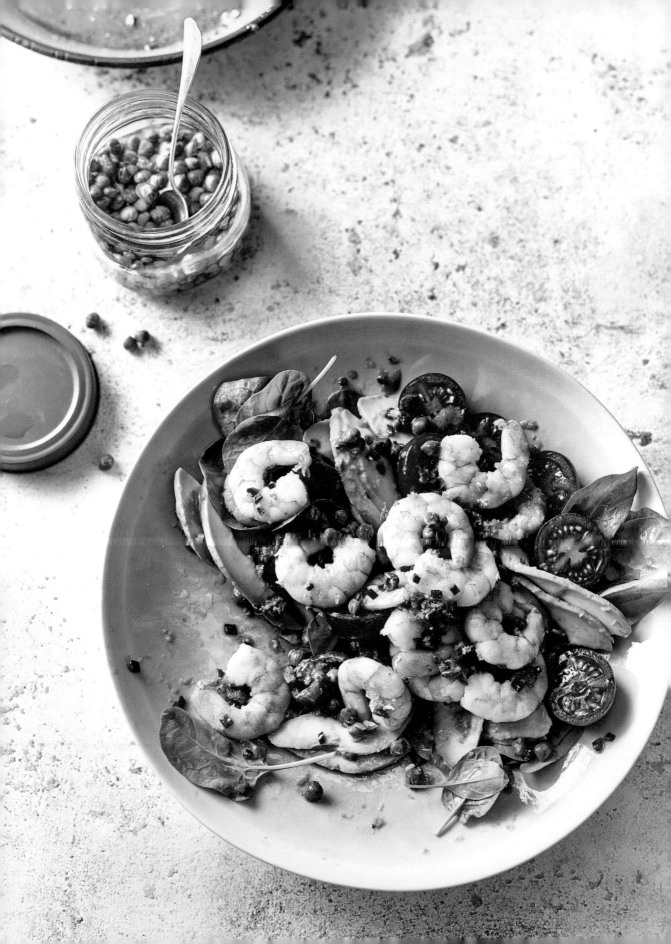

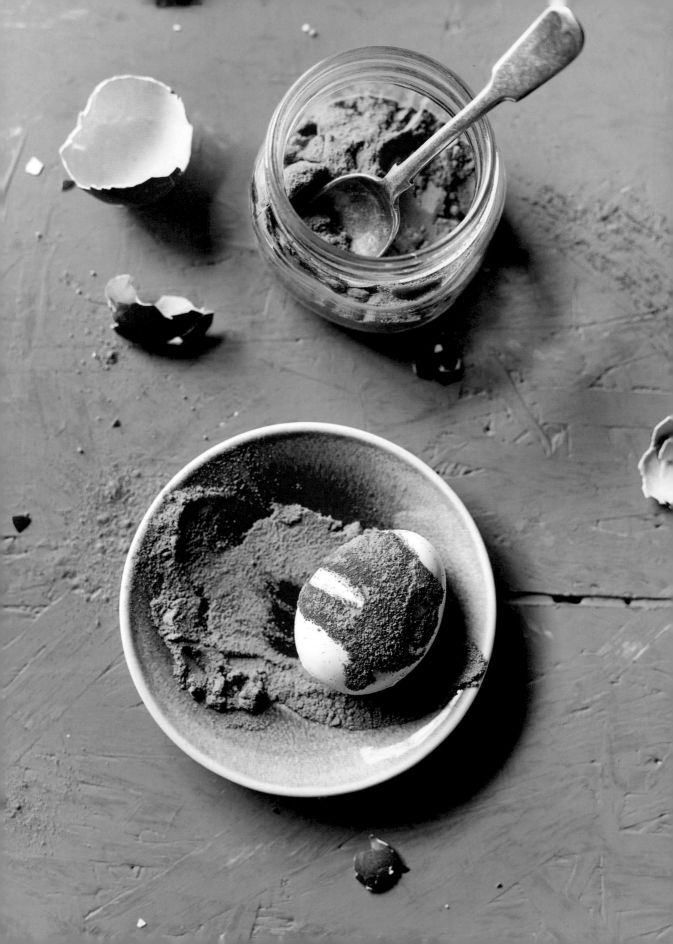

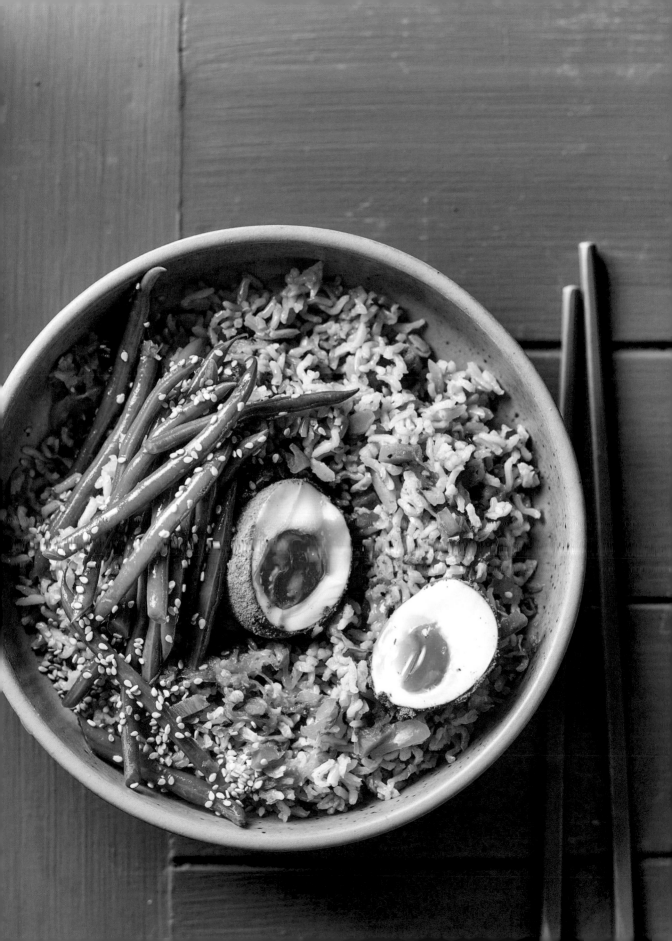

KIMCHI RICE WITH GREEN BEANS & TURMERIC SOFT-BOILED EGG

Kimchi is well known for containing healthy bacteria and probiotics that are so good for the gut. It's also low in calories and unbelievably tasty. You hardly need any other ingredients to make this nutritious dish shine; it's an awesome all-rounder for any time of the year.

Bring a medium pan of salted water to the boil and add the rice. Cook for 20 minutes or according to the packet instructions.

Meanwhile, bring a smaller pan of water to the boil and blanch the beans for 4 minutes. Remove from the water and set aside.

Bring a third pan of water to the boil, place the egg gently in the water and cook for 7 minutes. Run the egg under cold water and set aside.

Drain the cooked rice and put into a bowl. Mix the kimchi through the rice.

Heat the olive oil in a frying pan and sauté the green beans for a few minutes. Sprinkle over the sesame seeds and stir to coat.

Put the turmeric onto a small plate. Peel the boiled egg and roll the egg in turmeric, turning it to coat it all over.

Make a small well in the centre of the kimchi rice in the bowl and place the egg in the well. Add the sesame green beans on top.

Serves 1

100g (½ cup) brown rice
50g (1¾oz) green beans
1 egg
50g (3 tbsp) kimchi, chopped
1 tsp olive oil
1 tsp sesame seeds
1 tsp ground turmeric
sea salt

HERITAGE TOMATO SALAD WITH CARAMELIZED PEACHES, MOZZARELLA & OLIVES

Summer on a plate. Buy the tastiest tomatoes you can afford and make sure to use sweet, ripe peaches. You'll get a good dose of protein from the mozzarella.

Chop and slice the tomatoes in different ways so you get a variety of different shapes and sizes and place in a large bowl.

Season with salt and pepper, drizzle with the olive oil and balsamic vinegar and mix well. Set aside so the tomatoes can soak up the dressing.

Slice the peach into quarters and caramelize in a dry pan over a medium heat for 3–4 minutes, turning regularly.

Add the olives, mozzarella and basil to the bowl with the tomatoes and mix well.

When the peach quarters are nicely golden brown, place them on top of the salad and serve.

Serves 1

200g (7oz) heritage tomatoes
1 tbsp olive oil
1 tsp balsamic vinegar
1 peach, quartered
20g (¾oz) olives, sliced
50g (1¾oz) mozzarella, torn
1 bunch of basil, finely chopped
sea salt and freshly ground black pepper

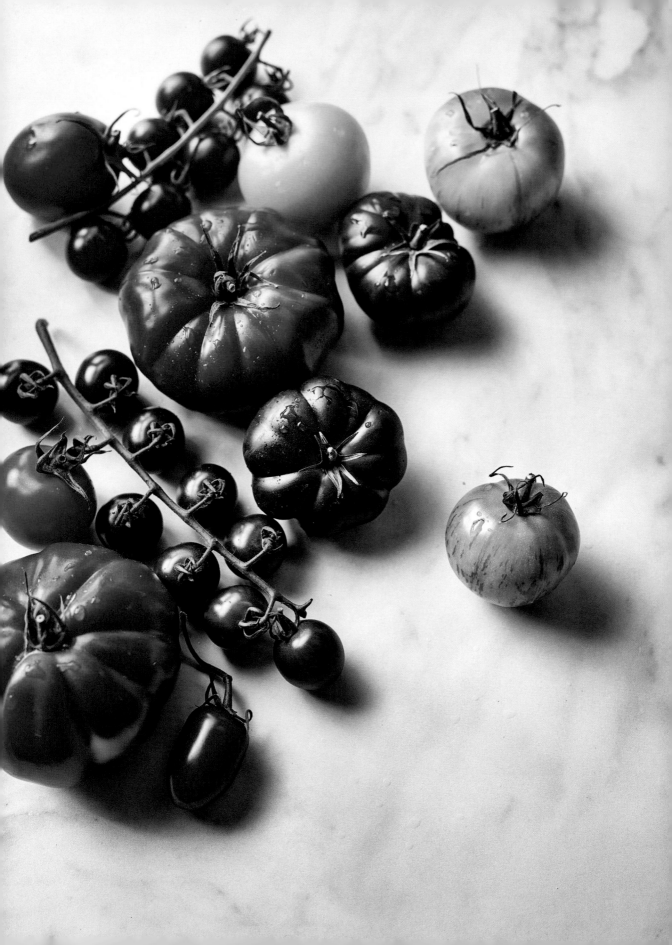

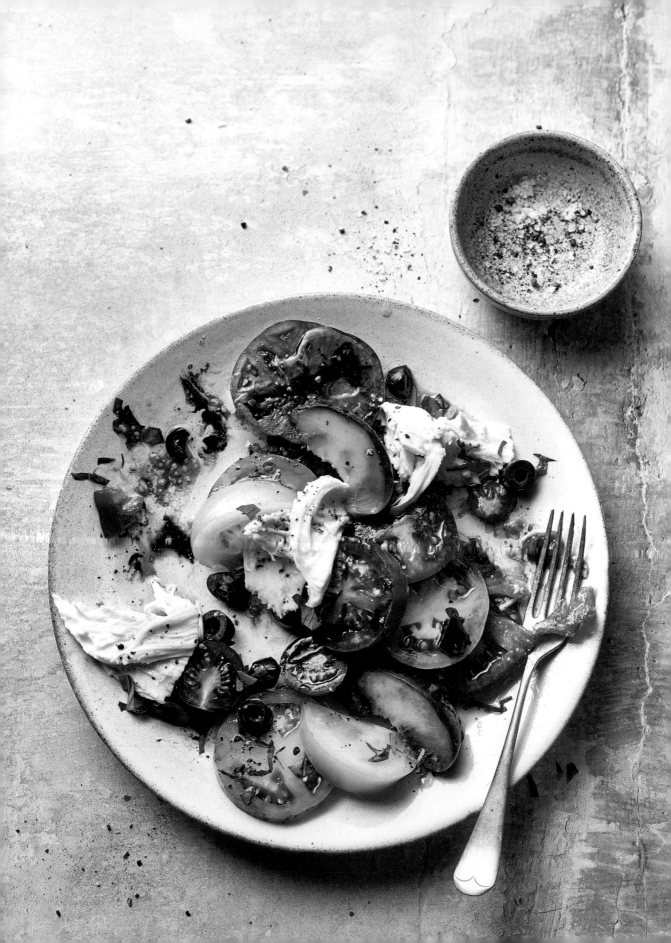

JERUSALEM ARTICHOKE SOUP WITH POACHED EGGS & SAUTEED MUSHROOMS

This is such a comforting soup that I recommend making double or triple quantities and freezing the leftovers in single portions for a rainy day. Jerusalem artichoke is full of protein and fibre and good for gut health.

Preheat the oven to 180°C/350°F/gas mark 4.

Place the Jerusalem artichokes on a baking tray and bake for 35–45 minutes or until they are soft when you stick a sharp knife in them.

Meanwhile, heat a little oil in a frying pan and sauté the mushrooms until nicely coloured. Season with salt and finish with a squeeze of lemon. Remove from the heat and set aside.

Once the artichokes are fully cooked, remove from the oven, roughly chop and transfer to a food processor. Blend until smooth, gradually adding the vegetable stock. Season with salt.

Poach the eggs. Fill a medium pan with water and bring to the boil. Add the vinegar, turn the heat down to a rolling boil and crack the eggs in, giving the water a slight stir.

Remove the eggs from the pan after 3–4 minutes using a slotted spoon and place them in the bottom of a deep soup bowl. Add the mushrooms, then pour over the hot soup.

Serves 1

200g (7oz) Jerusalem artichokes
½ tbsp olive oil
100g (3½oz) Paris brown mushrooms, sliced
½ lemon
200ml (¾ cup) vegetable stock
2 eggs
1 tbsp white wine vinegar
sea salt

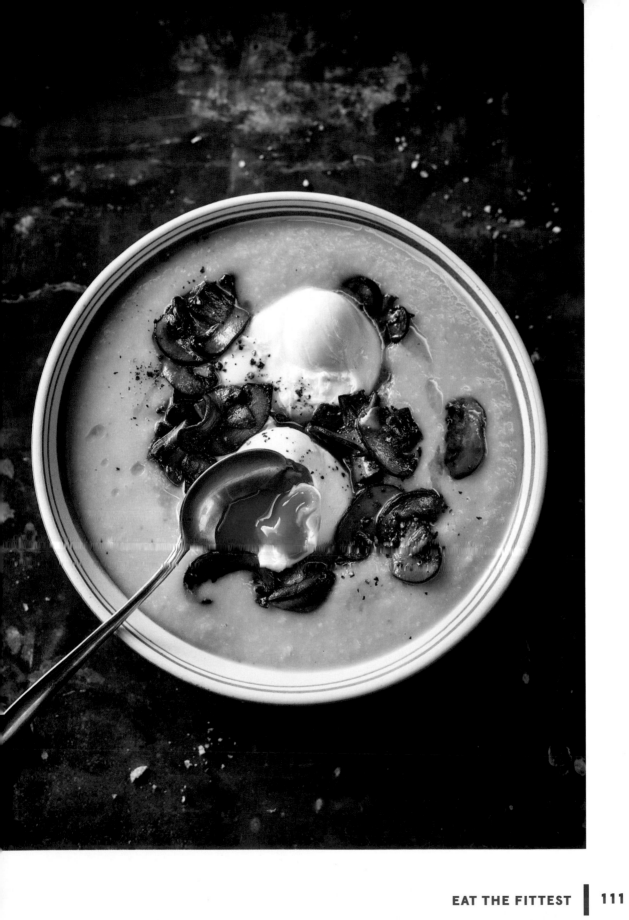

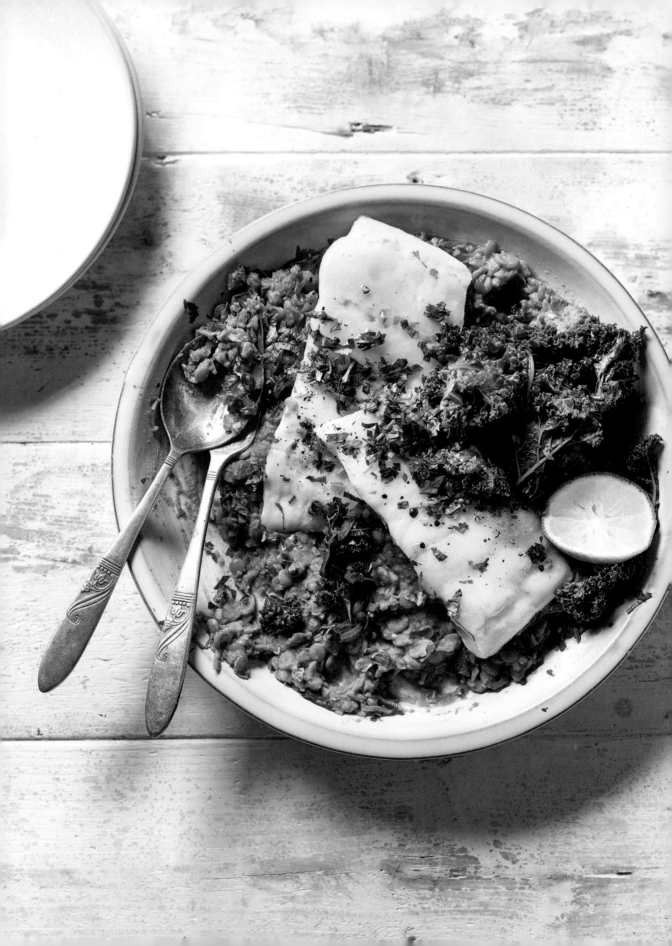

STEAMED HAKE WITH GREEN LENTIL DHAL & KALE

Steaming is one of the healthiest ways to cook fish, as it retains all the valuable nutrients. Lentils are a sound source of protein and iron. Put it all together with ginger, turmeric, chilli and fresh coriander and you've got an amazing dinner.

Soak the lentils in cold water overnight or for at least 2 hours. Preheat the oven to 140°C/300°F/gas mark 2.

First, make the dhal. In a food processor, blend the ginger, garlic, chilli powder, onion and turmeric to a paste.

Heat 1 tsp of the olive oil in a frying pan over a low heat. Add the paste and cook for a few minutes.

Add the soaked and drained lentils along with 3 times their volume of water (about 400ml/14 cups), the tomatoes and garam masala and bring to the boil, then turn down to a low heat. Simmer until the lentils have soaked up all the water and are starting to fall apart, about 20–25 minutes. Check for seasoning.

Meanwhile, cook the hake. Take some baking paper and lay on a baking tray. Place the hake on it with the remaining olive oil and salt and bake in the oven for 20–25 minutes.

Bring a pan of salted water to the boil and blanch the kale for 4 minutes.

Put the lentil dhal in a bowl and place the cooked fish on top. Sprinkle with the coriander (cilantro) and finish with the kale on top. Add a squeeze of lime and serve.

Serves 2

115g (⅝ cup) green lentils
1cm (½in) piece of fresh ginger
1 garlic clove
1 tsp chilli powder
1 small onion, roughly chopped
1cm (½in) piece of fresh turmeric
2 tsp olive oil
100g (3½oz) ripe tomatoes, chopped
pinch of garam masala
300g (10½oz) hake fillets
200g (7oz) kale, chopped
½ bunch of coriander (cilantro),
  finely chopped
½ lime
sea salt

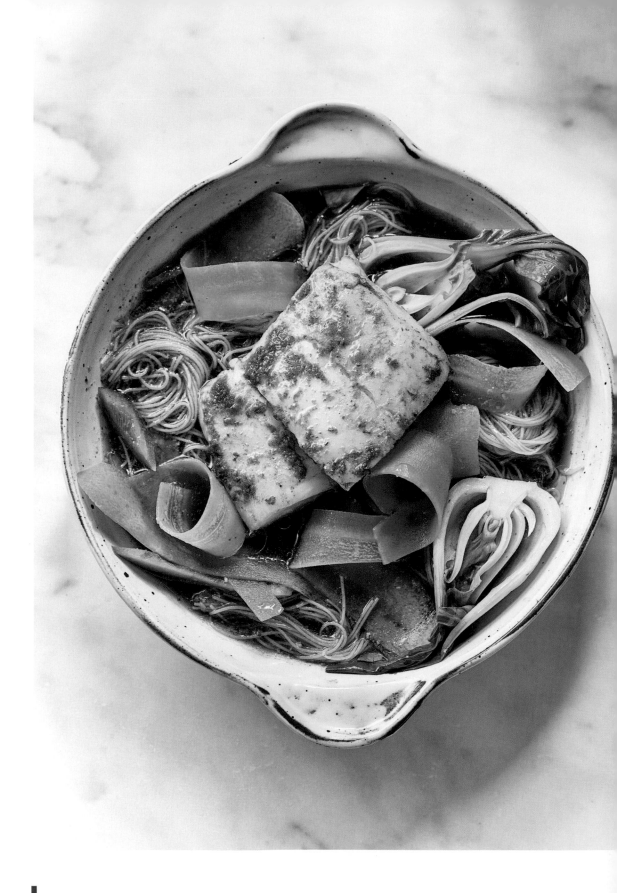

SPICED MARINATED COD WITH NOODLE BROTH & RAW VEG

It's worth marinating the cod here because it'll make it taste extra good. Keeping the vegetables raw allows them to retain all their nutrients.

Start by making the marinade for the cod. Use a pestle and mortar (or a blender if you don't have them). Add the coriander seeds, the fresh coriander (cilantro), the lime zest and juice, chilli and ginger and crush to a paste. Add 1 tsp of the honey and stir to combine.

Rub half of this onto your cod and leave to marinate in the fridge for 1 hour.

Preheat the oven to 190°C/375°F/gas mark 5. Line a baking tray with baking paper.

For the broth, add 250ml (1 generous cup) water to a pan on the stove over a medium heat. Add the miso and the remaining 1 tsp honey and season to taste with the soy sauce. Bring to the boil, then simmer for 5 minutes.

Remove the cod from the fridge, place on the lined baking tray and bake for 12–15 minutes.

Peel the carrot and discard the peel, then continue to peel the carrot into a bowl, so you have ribbons.

Bring a small pan of water to the boil and cook the noodles for 4–5 minutes or according to the packet instructions.

Once the fish is cooked, remove from the oven. Add the rest of the marinade to the simmering broth, stir well, then add the carrot ribbons, the (bell) pepper and pak choi (bok choy). Check the seasoning.

Place the noodles in a bowl and pour the broth over. Top with the fish and enjoy!

Serves 1

1 tsp coriander seeds
handful of chopped coriander (cilantro)
zest and juice of 1 lime
1 green chilli, finely chopped, deseeded (to taste)
2.5cm (1in) fresh ginger, peeled and chopped
2 tsp honey
150g (5¼oz) cod
1 tbsp miso paste
soy sauce
1 carrot
50g (1¾oz) rice noodles
1 green (bell) pepper, sliced
1 pak choi (bok choy), chopped

MISO-ROASTED CAULIFLOWER WITH KALE PESTO & CHERRY TOMATOES

This is a veggie superstar for when you crave a meat-free meal. Miso paste is a powerhouse of B vitamins, minerals and good bacteria for the gut, and so flavoursome. The almonds in the pesto are one of the best nuts to eat as they contain fibre, magnesium and healthy fats.

Soak the lentils in cold water overnight or for at least 2 hours.

Preheat the oven to 220°C/425°F/gas mark 7. Line a baking tray with baking paper.

Bring a pan of water to the boil, add the soaked and drained lentils and simmer for 20–25 minutes.

Mix the miso with a small amount of coconut oil to make a paste. Grate in the garlic cloves and mix well. Rub the paste all over the cauliflower.

Place the cauliflower on the lined baking tray and roast in the oven for 20 minutes.

To make the pesto, add the kale to a food processor. Cut the lemon in half and squeeze the juice from one of the halves over the kale. Add the almonds and a pinch of salt. Blend. Drizzle in the olive oil gradually until you have a paste-like texture. Add a little more lemon juice if necessary.

Drain the cooked lentils.

Remove the cauliflower from the oven. The outside should be nice and dark and caramelized.

Cut the cauliflower into florets and place in a bowl. Drizzle over the pesto, then sprinkle over the cherry tomatoes and add the lentils on top. Finish with a final squeeze of lemon.

Serves 1

100g (½ cup) green lentils
50g (1¾oz) white miso paste
1 tsp coconut oil
2 garlic cloves
1 cauliflower, leaves removed
100g (3½oz) kale, roughly chopped
1 lemon
20g (¾oz) almonds
1 tbsp olive oil
50g (1¾oz) cherry tomatoes, quartered
sea salt

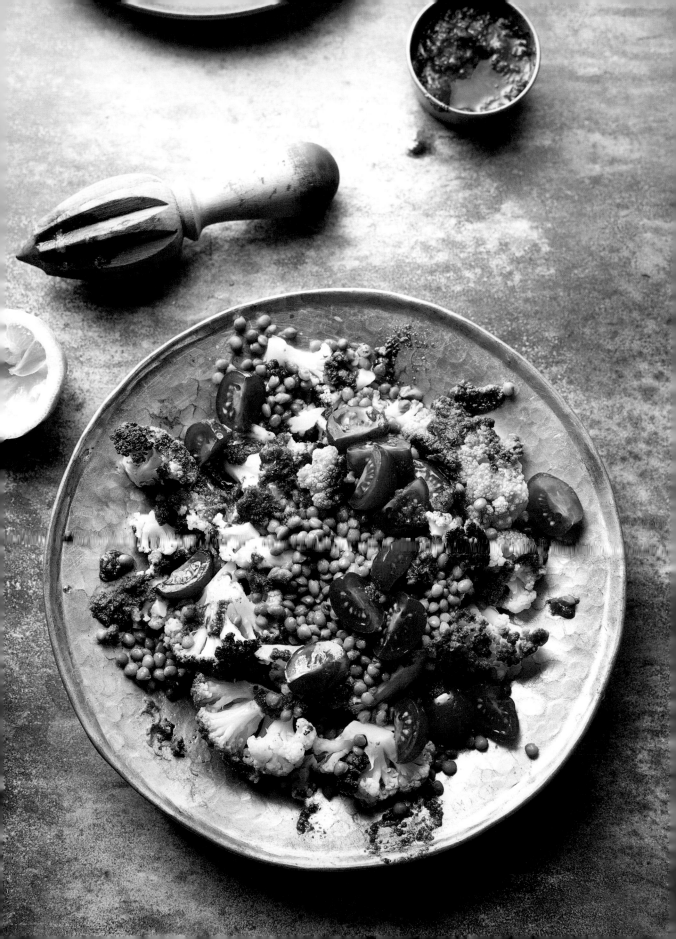

COUSCOUS WITH PEPPERS, BROCCOLI, CAPERS, PINE NUTS & ALMONDS

Vg

After a morning workout, couscous can be your much-needed lunchtime carbs. Broccoli, red pepper, capers, sultanas, pine nuts and almonds cap it all off for a perfectly balanced meal.

Place the couscous in a bowl with a pinch of salt. Pour over 100ml (generous ⅓ cup) boiling water. Add a drizzle of olive oil and leave to absorb for 10 minutes.

Heat 2 tbsp olive oil in a frying pan, add the curry powder and cook for 1 minute, then remove from the heat and allow to cool.

Add the capers, sultanas and pine nuts to the curry oil and mix well.

Heat a little more oil in a frying pan, add the broccoli and cook for 5–6 minutes until it is charred.

Sprinkle the almonds into the pan with the broccoli, finish with a squeeze of lemon and a pinch of salt.

Fluff up the couscous grains with a fork. Pour the curry dressing over the couscous and mix well. Add the (bell) pepper, then transfer to a plate and place the charred broccoli and almonds on top.

Serves 1

100g (⅔ cup) couscous
2–3 tbsp olive oil
1 tsp curry powder
10g (1 tbsp) capers
20g (¾oz) golden sultanas
10g (1 tbsp) pine nuts, toasted
100g (3½oz) Tenderstem broccoli
20g (¾oz) almonds, toasted and chopped
½ lemon
1 red (bell) pepper, diced
sea salt

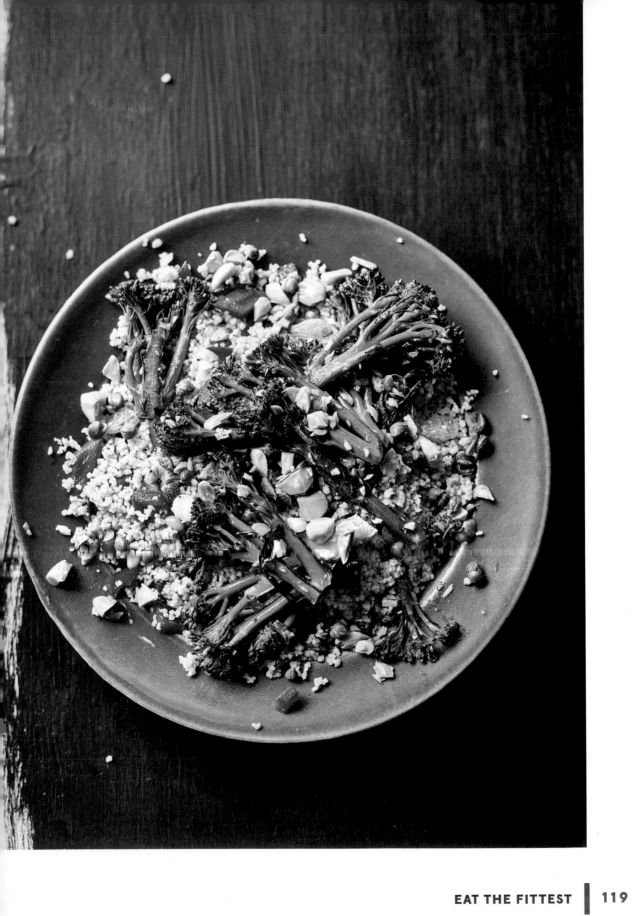

BAKED PAPRIKA CHICKEN WITH BROWN RICE

This is a bit of a heavier high-protein meal for that big hunger. I make this when I'm training hard every day and I want to keep my muscles fed with protein and my energy up. Good fuel.

Preheat the oven to 180°C/350°F/gas mark 4.

Add the olive oil to a frying pan over a medium heat. Add the chicken and cook, turning, for 8–10 minutes until starting to brown nicely. Transfer the chicken to a roasting pan, leaving as much oil behind in the pan as possible.

In the same pan, fry the onion for 10–12 minutes until softened and starting to caramelize, then add the paprika and tomato paste (purée) and stir to coat.

Add the stock to the pan, stir and bring to the boil. Pour the sauce over the chicken.

Put the chicken into the oven and bake for 45 minutes. Ten minutes before the end of cooking, add the spinach leaves, red (bell) pepper and olives to the roasting pan around the chicken and finish cooking.

Meanwhile, bring a pan of water to the boil and cook the brown rice according to the packet instructions.

Remove the chicken, spinach, peppers and olives from the oven and serve with the rice.

Serves 2

1 tbsp olive oil
2 chicken breasts or 4 boneless thighs – with skin for more flavour and fat, or skinless if you prefer
1 red onion, diced
4 tbsp paprika, or to taste
1 tsp tomato paste (purée)
570ml (2½ cups) chicken stock
2 big handfuls of baby spinach
2 roasted red (bell) peppers from a jar, roughly chopped
small handful of black olives
100g (½ cup) brown rice

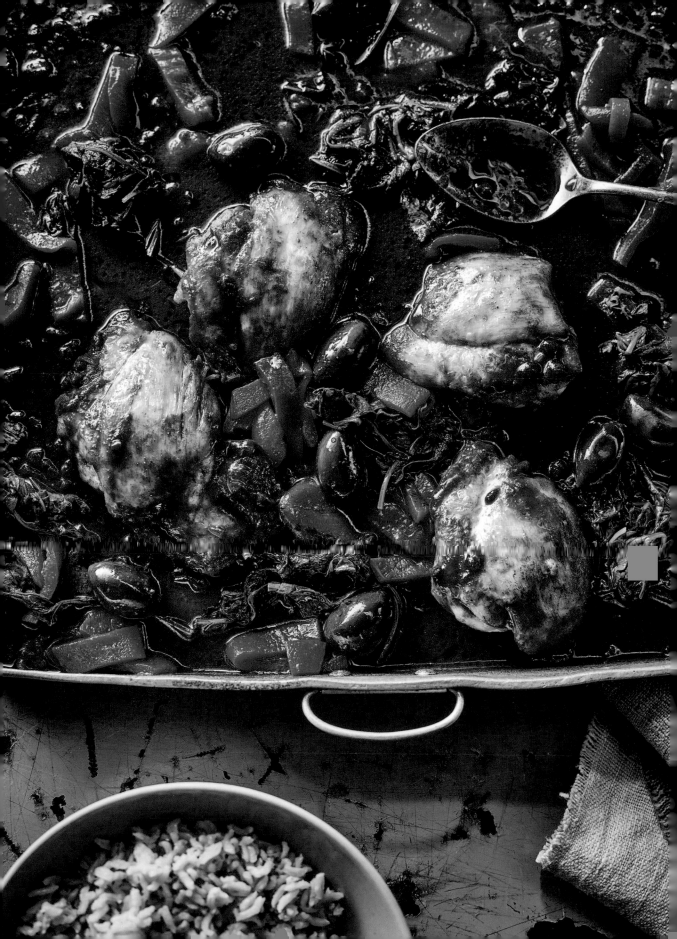

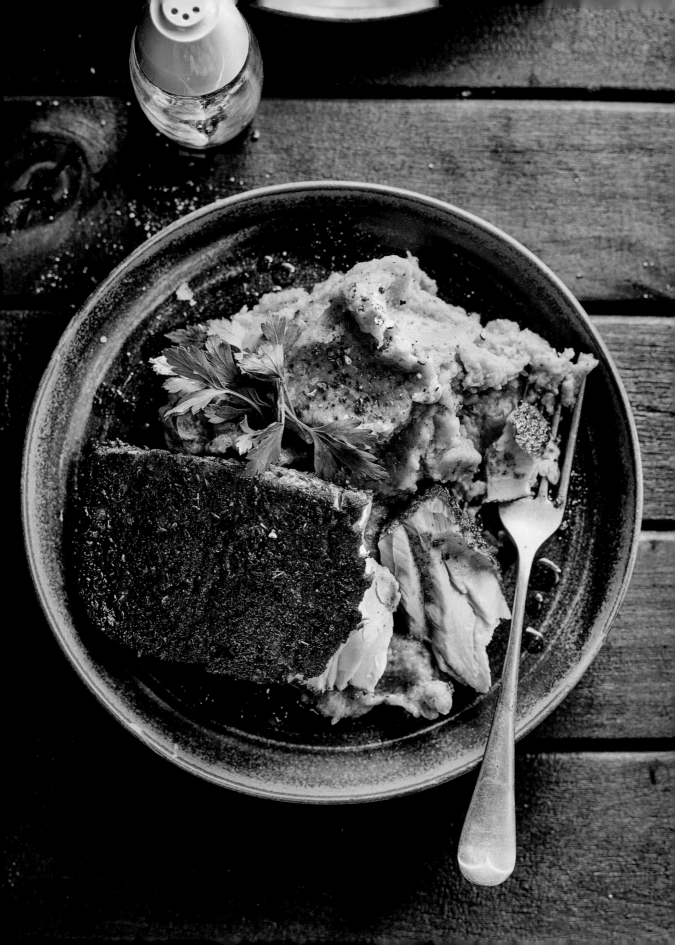

BLACKENED SALMON WITH SWEET POTATO, CARROT & BROCCOLI MASH

Here's another well-rounded meal and another favourite of mine. The mixed mash contains so much goodness and complements the salmon. There's a bit of a kick from the cayenne, paprika and chilli.

Preheat the oven to 160°C/325°F/gas mark 3.

In a small bowl, mix the paprika, cayenne pepper, cumin, parsley, garlic powder, chilli, oregano and a pinch of salt and pepper.

Brush the salmon fillets on both sides with the oil and roll in the spices until the whole fillet is evenly covered.

In a large, heavy frying pan over a high heat, cook the salmon, mixture side down, until blackened, 2–3 minutes, then turn over and cook the other side for the same length of time.

Add the vegetables, ½ tsp salt and enough water to cover the vegetables by at least 2.5cm (1in) to a large pot over a medium-high heat.

Bring to the boil and cook until the vegetables are tender, 10–15 minutes.

Transfer the salmon to a baking tray and cook in the oven for another 7–10 minutes.

Drain the vegetables and transfer to a large bowl with a splash of coconut milk. Mash using a potato masher until no lumps remain, then season well to taste.

Remove the salmon fillets from the oven and serve with the mash.

Serves 1

1 tsp paprika
¼ tsp cayenne pepper
1 tsp ground cumin
1 tbsp chopped fresh parsley
1 tsp garlic powder
½ fresh chilli, chopped, or ½–1 tsp dried chilli flakes
1 tsp dried oregano
1 salmon fillet, skinless or with skin, as preferred
1 tbsp coconut oil (or any oil of preference)
½ sweet potato, peeled and cubed
1 carrot, sliced
big handful of broccoli pieces
a little coconut milk, for the mash
sea salt and freshly ground black pepper

BAKED SWEET POTATO WITH TUNA, CHILLI & LIME

If you need evening energy, give this a go. The tuna and sweet potato are sustaining without being heavy. Lime makes it fresh and slightly sour; red onion gives sweetness; crème fraîche adds creaminess – perfectly balanced flavours.

Preheat the oven to 190°C/375°F/gas mark 5.

Prick the skin of the sweet potato all over with a fork. Place on a baking sheet and cook in the oven for around 50 minutes (or until tender).

Just before the potato is ready, heat the coconut oil in a frying pan and add the spinach. Cook for a few minutes until the leaves are wilted. Season with salt and pepper.

Remove the sweet potato from the oven and cut it in half lengthways. Scatter the tuna on top of both halves. Next, add the red onion and chilli (if using) on top of the tuna.

Cut the lime in half and generously squeeze the juice all over. Cut the remaining lime into slices. Garnish the dish with the fresh coriander (cilantro) and lime slices, and serve with the crème fraîche, black pepper, and the wilted spinach.

Serves 1

1 sweet potato (approx 200g/7oz)
1 tbsp coconut oil
2 large handfuls of baby spinach
1 x 145g (5oz) can tuna in spring water, drained
½ red onion, finely sliced
1 red chilli, finely sliced (optional)
1 lime
2 tbsp chopped fresh coriander (cilantro)
3 tbsp crème fraîche
sea salt and freshly ground black pepper

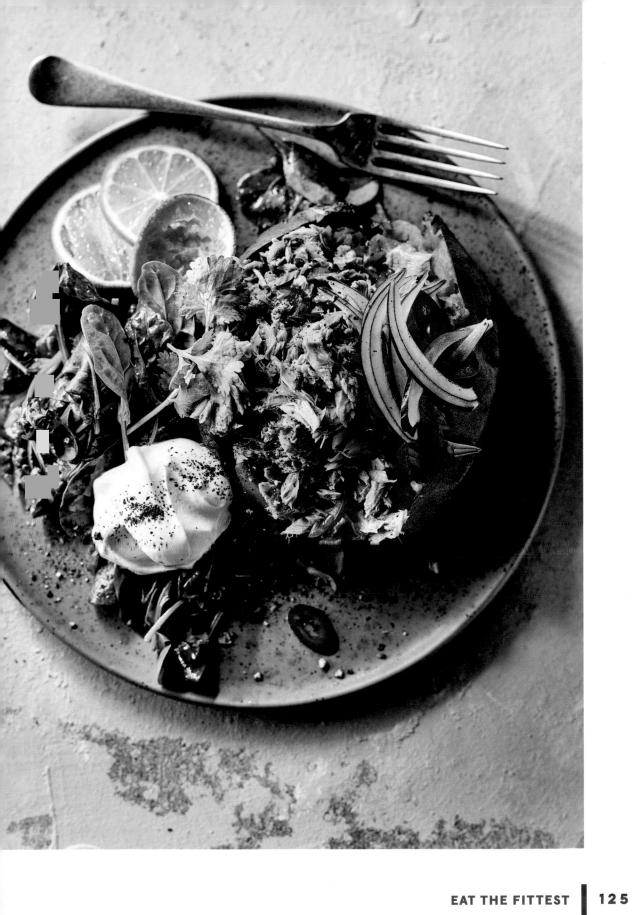

AUBERGINE & TOFU CURRY WITH BROWN RICE

Vg

Aubergines are rich in antioxidants – thanks to their purple skin – as well as dietary fibre and magnesium. Tofu is a great vegetarian protein, is versatile and takes on flavours really well. If you're suspicious of aubergine and tofu, promise me you'll try this dish; I guarantee you will be converted!

Heat the coconut oil in a frying pan over a medium heat and add the aubergine (eggplant). Gently fry for 8–10 minutes.

Add the onion, tofu, garlic and ginger and season with salt. Cook for a further 5 minutes, then add the curry powder. Stir to combine.

Add the vegetable stock and bring to the boil, then simmer gently for 10–15 minutes.

Put the brown rice into a pan with half the coconut milk. Top up with 200ml (¾ cup) water and cook for 20 minutes.

Add the remaining coconut milk to the curry and cook for a further 5–10 minutes or until the sauce has slightly thickened. Serve the curry with the cooked, drained rice and finish with a squeeze of fresh lime juice. Garnish with fresh coriander (cilantro).

Serves 2

1 tbsp coconut oil
1 aubergine (eggplant), cut into 2.5cm (1in) cubes
1 onion, finely diced
150g (5¼oz) silken tofu, cubed
1 garlic clove, chopped
2.5cm (1in) fresh ginger, chopped
2 tbsp curry powder
100ml (generous ⅓ cup) vegetable stock
100g (½ cup) brown rice
1 x 400ml (14fl oz) can coconut milk
1 lime
fresh coriander (cilantro)
sea salt

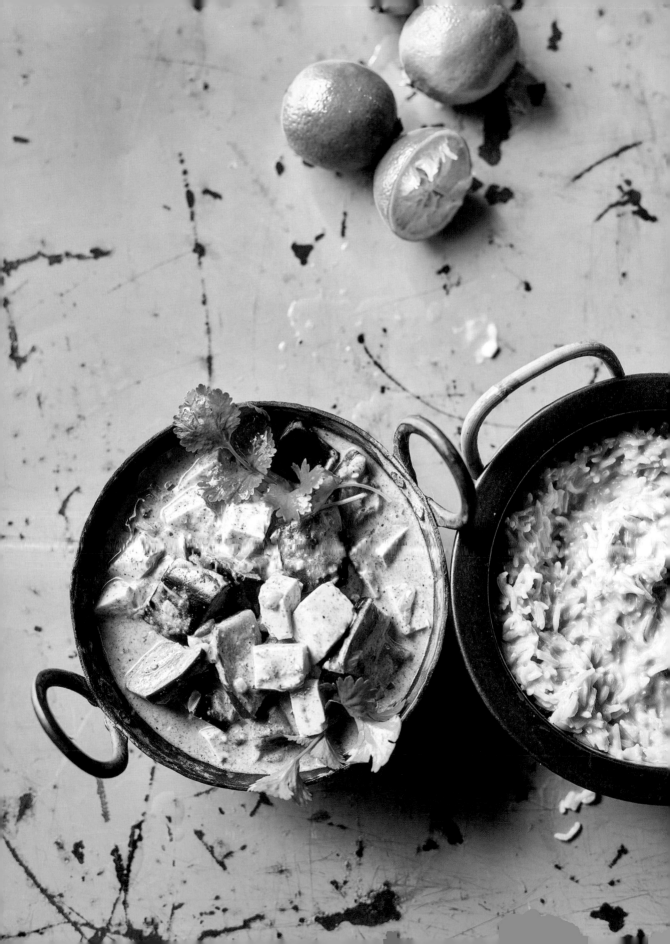

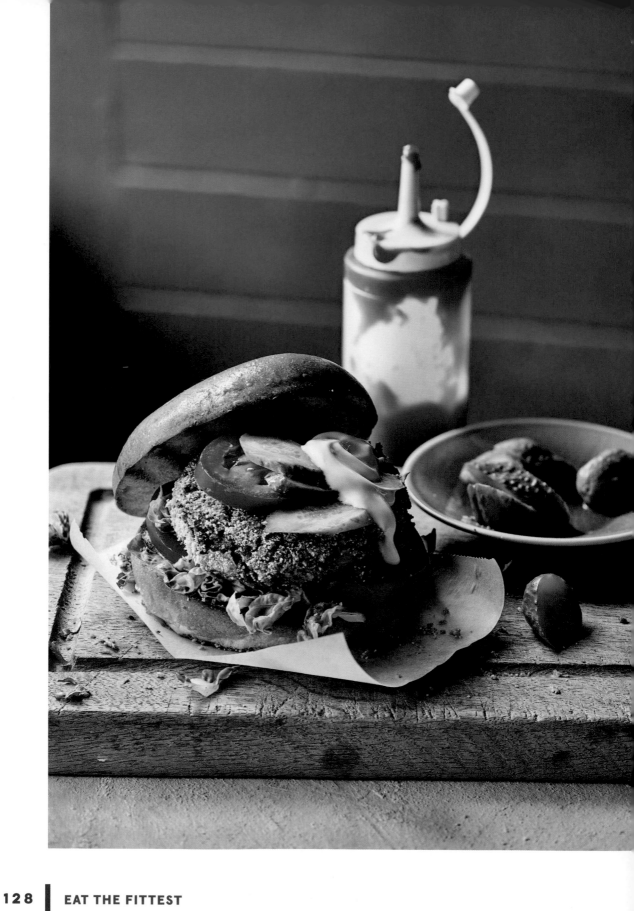

VEGAN FULL-OF-BEANS BURGER

To really replicate the texture of a beef burger, don't blitz the beans too much in the food processor – you want some texture in there. When you add a burger bun and all the extras, you'll have your favourite junk food with all the satisfaction and none of the junk.

Put the chickpeas (garbanzo beans), kidney beans and onion into a food processor and pulse a few times, but do not blend fully.

Add all the herbs and spices, salt and pepper, and mix well.

Using your hands, shape the mix into two balls.

Mix the flour and polenta (cornmeal) together. Roll the balls in the flour/polenta mix to coat them, and then press each one into a burger shape. Or use a burger press.

Heat the coconut oil in a frying pan over a medium heat and fry the burgers for 3–4 minutes on each side, until golden brown.

Split the burger buns and toast the cut side of each half.

Place a burger on each of the bun bases, then layer with sliced gherkin, lettuce, sliced tomato and finally a dollop of coconut yogurt and ketchup.

Serves 2

100g (¾ cup) canned chickpeas
  (garbanzo beans)
100g (¾ cup) canned kidney beans
½ onion, finely chopped
1 tsp chopped fresh coriander (cilantro)
1 tsp chopped fresh parsley
½ red or green chilli, deseeded and chopped
1 tsp ground cumin
1 tsp paprika
½ tsp sea salt
1 tsp freshly ground black pepper
100g (¾ cup) rice flour
100g (¾ cup) polenta (cornmeal)
1 tsp coconut oil, for frying

To serve
2 vegan burger buns
1 gherkin, sliced
1 baby gem lettuce, sliced
1 tomato, sliced
1 tbsp coconut yogurt
1 tbsp tomato ketchup

MACKEREL, TOMATO & RED ONION RICE SALAD

Mackerel is an oily fish packed with omega-3 fatty acids that are believed to help your body repair after a workout and build muscle. With the brown rice, strong red onion, rich mackerel and fresh parsley, this is a flavour-packed, lean meal that's ideal after a workout.

Cook the brown rice according to the packet instructions.

Put the tomatoes, onion and parsley into a bowl with the vinegar. Season well and mix everything together.

Add the coconut oil to a frying pan over a medium-high heat and fry the mackerel pieces for 3-4 minutes. Make sure you make the mackerel as crispy as you can.

Once fried and nicely crispy, place the mackerel on a plate lined with kitchen paper, to soak up any excess oil.

Serve the mackerel on a plate, garnished with the tomato and onion salad.

Serves 1-2

50g (¼ cup) brown rice
2 large tomatoes, diced
½ red onion, finely diced
50g (1¾oz) chopped fresh parsley
2-3 tbsp apple cider vinegar
1 tbsp coconut oil
160g (5½oz) sweetcure smoked mackerel
sea salt and freshly ground black pepper

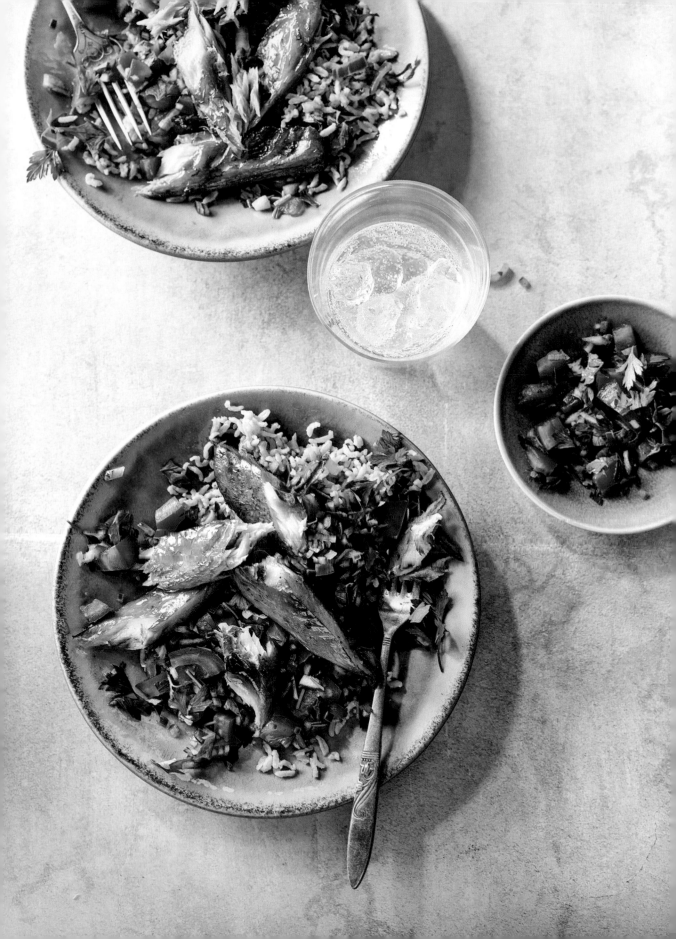

SPINACH, TOFU, CHICKPEA & POTATO CURRY

Vg

A wholesome vegan curry with potatoes, ginger, tofu and coconut to warm you up on a miserable day.

Heat the coconut oil in a frying pan over a medium heat and add the onion. Cook gently for about 8 minutes until starting to soften and caramelize.

Add the ginger and tofu to the pan with the curry powder and garam masala, stir to combine and cook for a further 2–3 minutes.

Add the chickpeas (garbanzo beans) and 50ml (3½ tbsp) of the liquid from the can of chickpeas. Simmer gently for 5 minutes.

Add the new potatoes to the curry. Cook for 2 minutes, then add the coconut milk. Simmer gently for a further 5 minutes.

Finally, add the spinach, stir through the sauce and allow it to wilt. Your curry sauce should be thick and glossy at this point. If it's not, allow it to reduce down further.

Meanwhile, steam the broccoli in a microwave or over a pan of simmering water until just tender.

Check the seasoning of the curry and serve with the steamed broccoli.

Serves 2

1 tbsp coconut oil
1 onion, finely diced
20g (¾oz) fresh ginger
300g (10½oz) silken tofu, cubed
20g (¾oz) curry powder
20g (¾oz) garam masala
½ x 400g (14oz) can chickpeas (garbanzo beans)
200g (7oz) cooked new potatoes, quartered
200ml (¾ cup) coconut milk
200g (7oz) baby spinach
½ head of broccoli, cut into pieces
sea salt and freshly ground black pepper

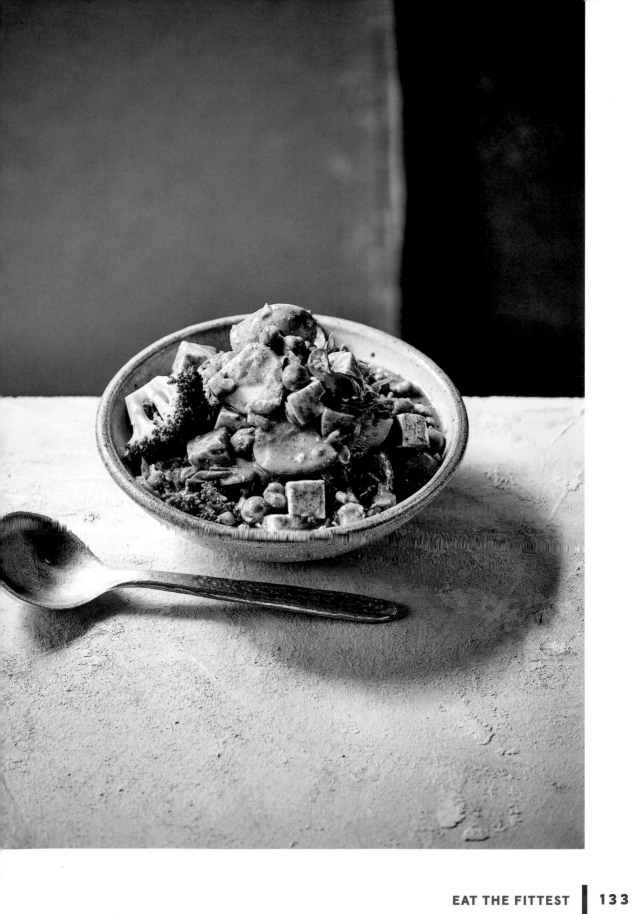

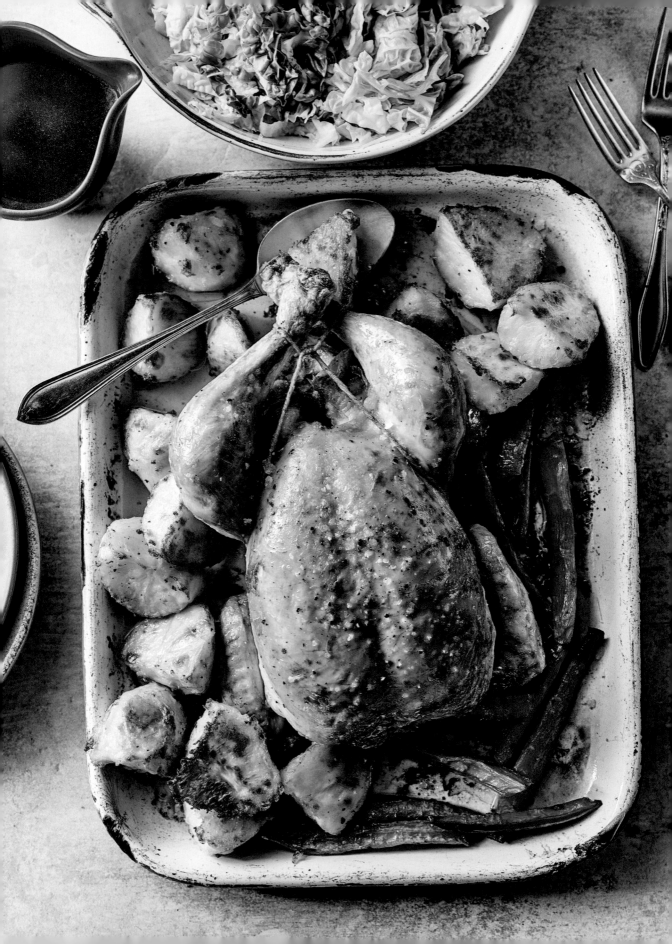

HEALTHIER ROAST CHICKEN & POTATOES WITH CABBAGE & CARROTS

It really is possible for the Sunday roast to be healthy and to please the whole family!

Preheat the oven to 220°C/425°F/gas mark 7.

Place the chicken on a baking tray (removing any giblets if necessary) and arrange the carrots around. Rub 1 tbsp olive oil all over the chicken, season all over with salt and pepper, and roast in the oven for 1½ hours.

Meanwhile, rinse the potatoes in cold water, place in a large saucepan and cover with water. Add a pinch of salt and place the pan over a high heat. Bring to the boil and allow to boil for 10 minutes.

About 40 minutes after you put the chicken in the oven, add 3 tbsp olive oil to a deep baking tray and place in the oven for 5 minutes to heat up. Drain the potatoes and return them to the pan. Fluff up the potatoes by tossing them around the pan and leave to steam dry. Remove the tray of hot oil from the oven and place the potatoes carefully into the oil. Cook for 30–40 minutes, turning occasionally, until golden and crisp.

When it's had its 1½ hours, remove the chicken from the oven and pierce a thick part of the flesh – if the juices run clear, it's cooked. If not, put back into the oven for a few more minutes. When it's ready, loosely cover with foil and rest for 15 minutes.

Bring the stock to the boil and add the cabbage. Cook gently for 10 minutes, then drain. Take the potatoes out of the oven.

Add the gravy to a pan with any chicken juices and heat through. Serve the chicken with the vegetables and gravy.

Serves 4

1 free-range whole chicken, about 1.3kg (2lb 14oz)
3 carrots, peeled and cut into large matchsticks
olive oil
4 baking potatoes, peeled and quartered
500ml (generous 2 cups) vegetable stock
½ Savoy cabbage, sliced
300ml (1¼ cups) store-bought chicken gravy
sea salt and freshly ground black pepper

DINNERS

GREEN PAPAYA & MISO AUBERGINE SALAD

Papaya helps digestion and contains antioxidants that fight inflammation. Paired with aubergine and this punchy dressing, it makes a sweet, salty, sour, spicy, rich plate of food.

Preheat the oven to 180°C/350°F/gas mark 4.

Cut the ends off the aubergine (eggplant), then cut into large cubes. Arrange the aubergine on a baking tray, drizzle over the coconut oil and toss well to coat all the pieces of aubergine. Place in the oven and bake for 25 minutes.

Mix the miso paste and balsamic vinegar together in a small bowl and season with salt and pepper. Set aside.

Remove the skin from the papaya and use a peeler (or grater) to peel the papaya flesh into ribbons in a bowl. Add the green beans.

Crush the garlic cloves in a pestle and mortar with the chilli(es), then put into a small bowl. Add the honey, fish sauce and lime juice and mix well. Pour the dressing over the papaya and beans and mix well. Add the tomatoes and crushed peanuts and mix everything together.

Remove the aubergine from the oven, add the miso mix and toss well to coat the pieces all over. Cook for a further 5 minutes, then remove from the oven.

Serve the dressed papaya salad on a plate with the aubergine on top.

Serves 2

1 aubergine (eggplant)
1 tbsp coconut oil, melted
2 tbsp miso paste
1 tsp balsamic vinegar
1 green papaya, halved and deseeded
100g (3½oz) green beans, roughly chopped into 5cm (2in) pieces
3 garlic cloves
1–2 small red chillies, finely chopped
1 tbsp honey
1 tsp fish sauce, depending on taste
juice of 1 lime
5 cherry tomatoes, quartered
2 tbsp peanuts, crushed
sea salt and freshly ground black pepper

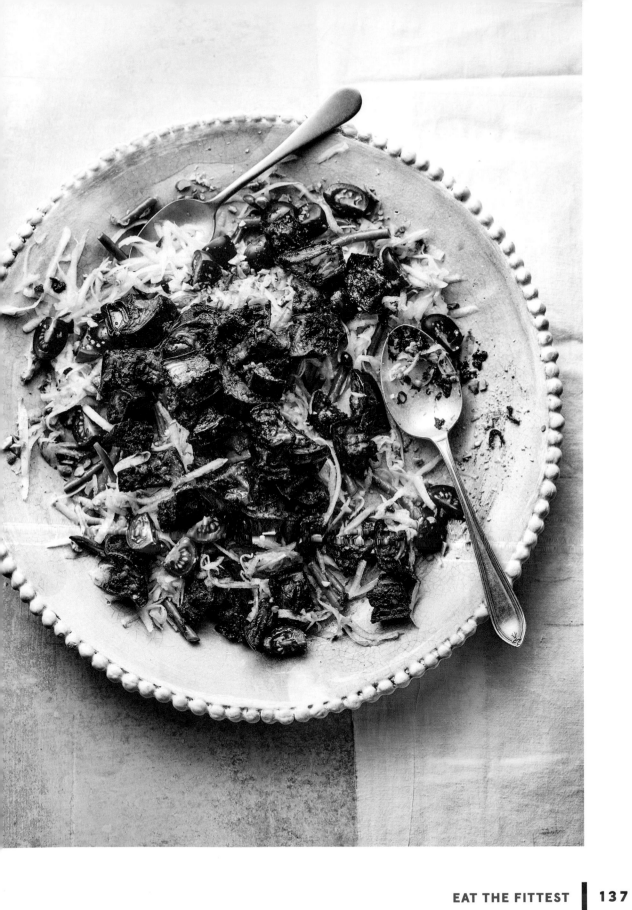

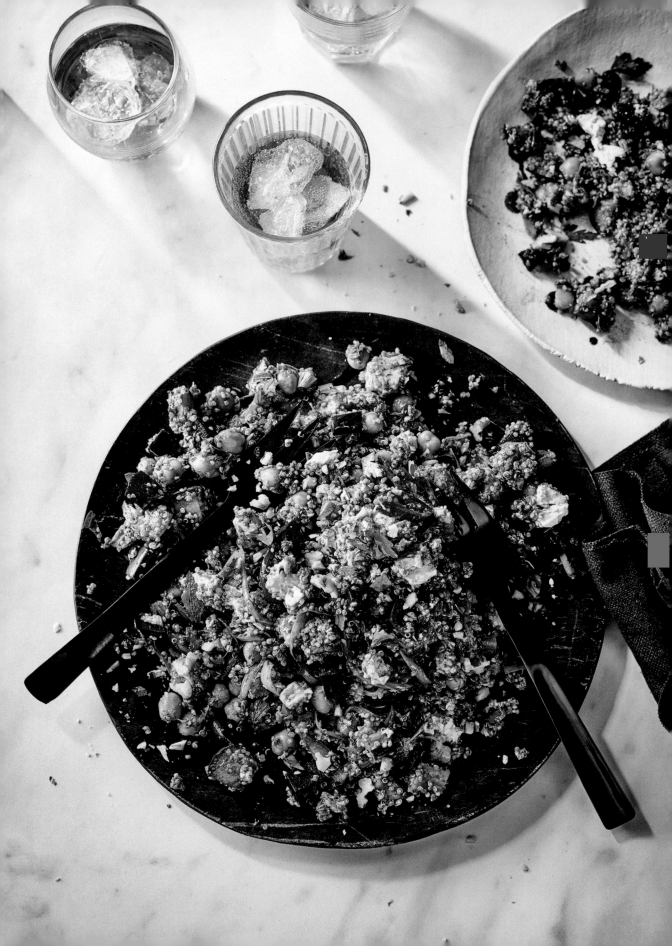

SUPERFOOD SALAD WITH QUINOA, TOFU, BEETROOT & AUBERGINE

Vg

You've probably heard that quinoa is a superfood! It's very high in fibre and contains all nine essential amino acids, making it a complete protein source. What's more, it's gluten-free. Cooked beetroot (plain, not in vinegar) is so useful to have in the fridge as it can be added to lots of salads. This is a super spring salad for dinner.

Rinse the quinoa in cold water. Put 150ml (⅔ cup) water into a saucepan, add the quinoa and bring to the boil. Simmer for about 12 minutes or until all the water has evaporated and the quinoa has doubled in size, then remove from the heat.

Meanwhile, put 2 tsp of the olive oil in a frying pan and add the onion and spices. Fry for 5–7 minutes until the onion has softened.

Add the garlic, chilli and tofu and fry for a further 2–3 minutes. Add the tomato paste (purée), season with salt and pepper, then add the chickpeas (garbanzo beans) and leave to simmer for 5 minutes.

Add the chopped beetroot to the cooked quinoa with the parsley and mix.

Fry the diced aubergine (eggplant) in the remaining 1 tsp olive oil for 5–6 minutes until softened and season with salt and pepper.

Transfer the spiced chickpeas and tofu to a bowl, then add the quinoa and beetroot and the aubergine and mix. Sprinkle over the walnuts and serve.

Serves 2–3

50g (¼ cup) quinoa
1 tbsp olive oil
1 onion, sliced
1 tsp curry powder
1 tsp ground cumin
1 tsp ground turmeric
1 tsp ground cinnamon
1 garlic clove, crushed
½ red or green chilli
100g (3½oz) silken tofu, cubed
1 tbsp tomato paste (purée)
½ x 400g (14oz) can chickpeas
  (garbanzo beans)
50g (1¾oz) cooked beetroot, chopped
1 tbsp chopped fresh parsley
1 aubergine (eggplant), diced
1 tbsp chopped walnuts
sea salt and freshly ground black pepper

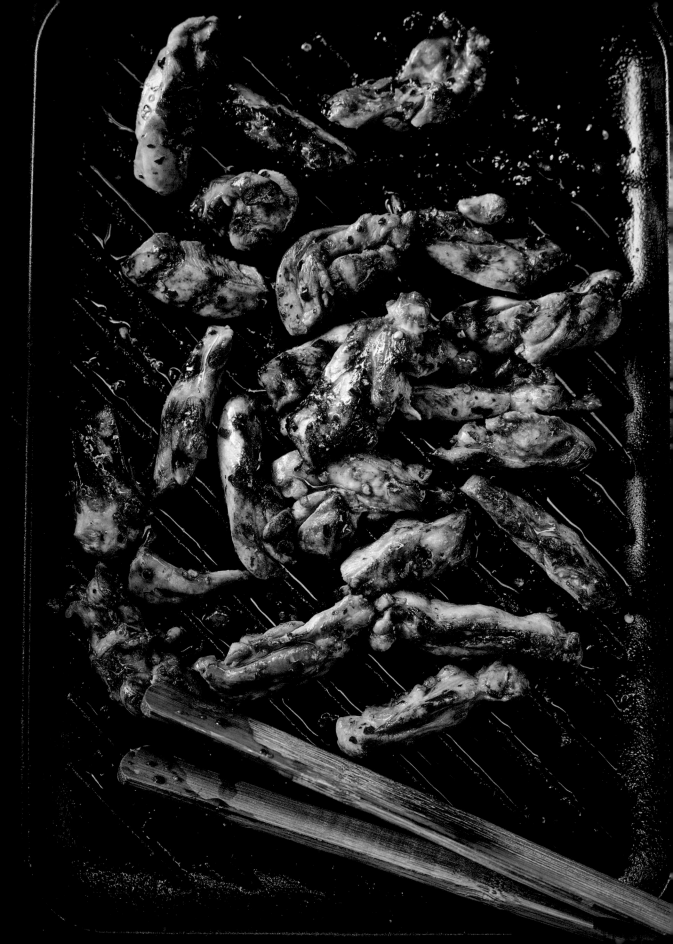

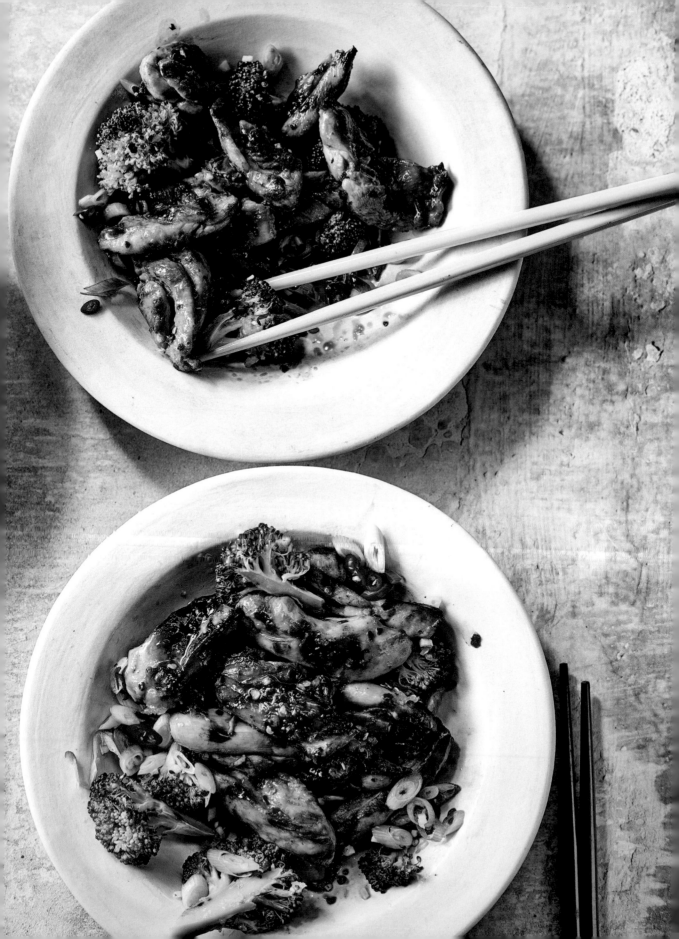

THE ULTIMATE CHICKEN SALAD

If you're looking for a new riff on salad, this is for you. Salad doesn't have to mean rabbit food! This ultimate chicken salad is substantial and delicious.

First, make the marinade. Put all the marinade ingredients into a large bowl and mix well. Add the chicken thighs and stir well so they are fully coated. Cover and refrigerate for at least 20 minutes or overnight.

When you are ready to start cooking, heat a griddle pan until very hot and remove the chicken from the marinade, reserving the marinade. Lightly char the chicken pieces on all sides in the pan for a couple of minutes.

Put the leftover marinade in a saucepan, bring to the boil, then simmer gently for 5 minutes. Add the charred chicken thighs and cook for a further 10–12 minutes until cooked through.

Heat a dry frying pan and cook the broccoli over a medium heat for about 7 minutes, tossing regularly.

Put the cooked broccoli, spring onions (scallions), garlic, ginger, chillies and lime juice in a bowl and mix well.

Serve the broccoli salad alongside the chicken and its sauce drizzled over the top.

Serves 2

4 skinless, boneless chicken thighs, sliced
½ head of broccoli, chopped into pieces
2 spring onions (scallions), finely chopped
2 garlic cloves, crushed
½ tsp finely chopped fresh ginger
2 small red or green chillies, finely chopped
juice of 2 limes

For the marinade
2 tbsp soy sauce
2 tbsp fish sauce
1 generous tbsp honey
1 garlic clove, crushed
2 crushed chillies
juice of 1 lime
1 tbsp coconut oil, melted

RICE BOWL WITH BROWN RICE, TOFU, GREENS & A POACHED EGG

V

If you're so exhausted you feel like you're at death's door, this will revive you! A mega nutritious meat-free meal in a bowl. It's got so much going for it.

Fold a few pieces of kitchen paper and place them on a cutting board. Put the tofu on top, then add another few folded pieces of kitchen paper. Put another small cutting board on top, and add a weight (a can, for example). Leave for 30 minutes until the moisture has been absorbed by the paper.

Cook the rice according to the packet instructions, then drain.

Meanwhile, boil another pan of water over a high heat, add the broccoli and kale and cook for 3–4 minutes. Drain and set aside.

Cut the tofu into cubes.

In a bowl, mix the sesame oil and soy sauce, then add the tofu and mix well to coat.

Heat the coconut oil in a frying pan. Remove the tofu from the marinade, shaking off any excess liquid and add to the pan. Cook for a few minutes, turning frequently, until golden.

Poach the egg. Fill a medium pan with water and bring to the boil. Add the vinegar, turn the heat down to a rolling boil and crack the egg in, giving the water a slight stir.

Remove the egg from the pan after 3–4 minutes using a slotted spoon.

Put the cooked rice into a serving bowl, then add the kale and broccoli. Sprinkle the tofu cubes over the top. Place the kimchi to one side of the bowl and the poached egg on the other side. Season with some salt and pepper and add a drizzle of sesame oil.

Serves 1

100g (3½oz) silken tofu
50g (¼ cup) brown rice
¼ head of broccoli, chopped into pieces
handful of kale leaves, torn
1 tbsp toasted sesame oil, plus extra for drizzling
2 tbsp soy sauce
1 tbsp coconut oil
1 egg
1 tbsp white wine vinegar
1 tbsp organic kimchi
sea salt and freshly ground black pepper

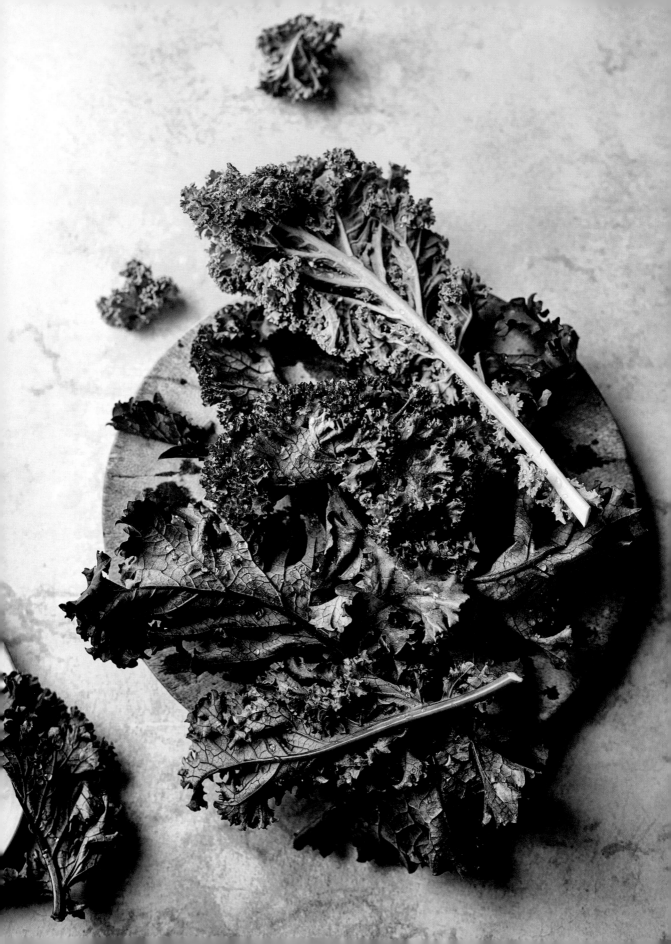

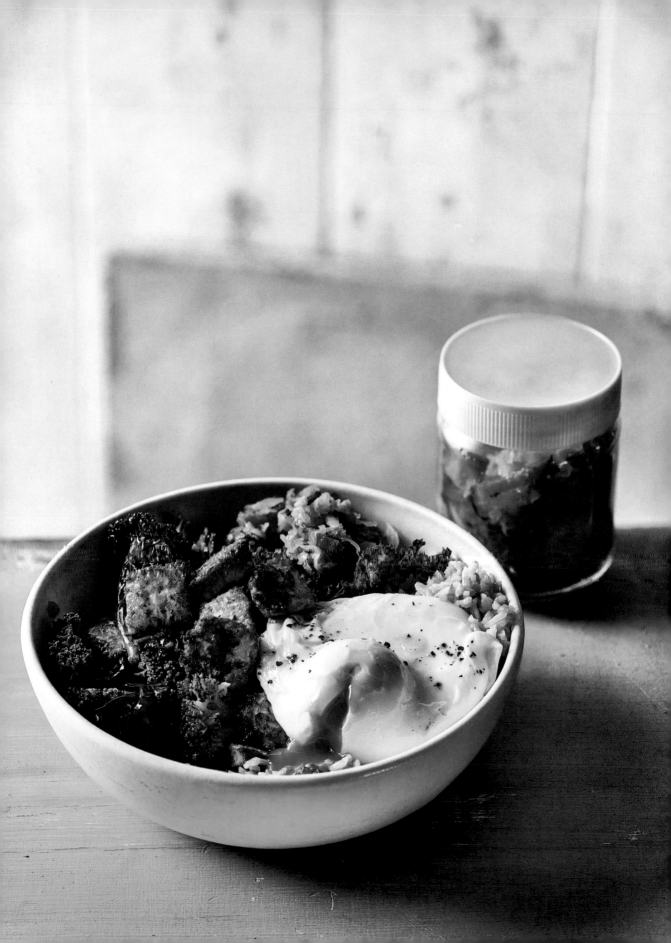

SUPER-EASY SUPER-FRESH BAKED SALMON PARCELS

This is like a taste of spring in one handy parcel. Cooking everything in a parcel with slices of lemon creates incredibly good juices and freshness. The asparagus will provide you with vitamins A, C, E and K.

Preheat the oven to 190°C/375°F/gas mark 5. Divide the asparagus, broccoli and tomatoes between two foil squares, placing them in the middle of each square, with a few lemon slices on top.

Sit the salmon fillets on the beds of the vegetables and lemon, then place more lemon slices on top of the salmon. Sprinkle the garlic, parsley and salt all over. Add 1 tbsp coconut oil to the top of each salmon fillet, then seal the foil parcels by folding up the edges. Place the parcels on a baking tray and cook for 20 minutes.

Remove from the oven and place each parcel on a plate to be opened at the table.

Serves 2

6 asparagus spears
6 pieces long-stem broccoli
10 cherry or small vine tomatoes
2 lemons, thinly sliced
2 skinless salmon fillets
2 garlic cloves, crushed
1 tsp chopped fresh parsley
pinch of sea salt
2 tbsp coconut oil

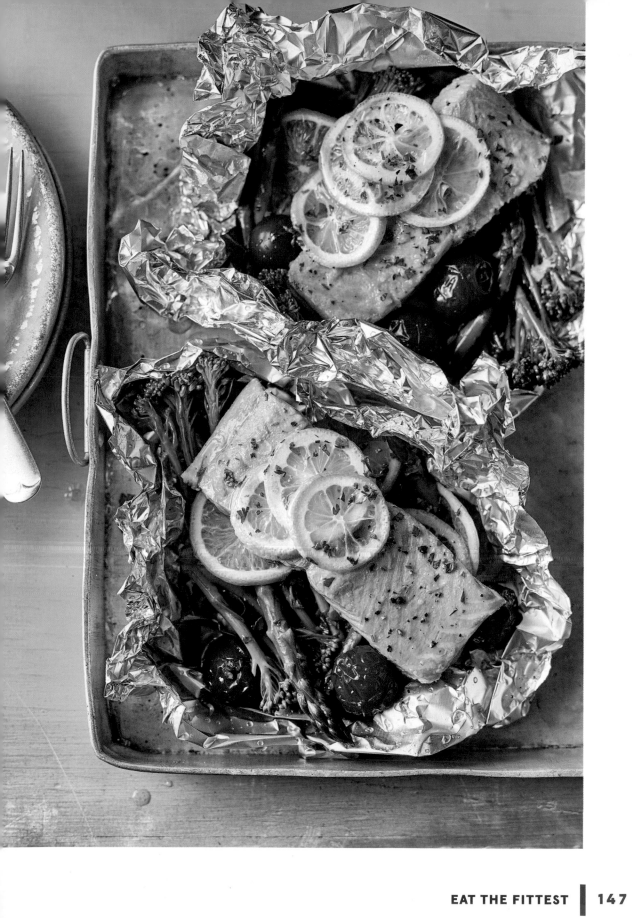

BE THE FITTEST MEDITERRANEAN SALAD

V

Doesn't this salad look amazing?! Pomegranate makes any plate of food look pretty and if your food looks good, it'll taste even better. If you're vegetarian, try to find a feta made without rennet, or substitute for a vegetarian equivalent.

Trim the bottom off the lettuce, then cut in half lengthwise and spread the leaves out flat on a plate.

Place the cucumber, tomatoes and red onion on top of the leaves and sprinkle over the feta. Top with the parsley and pomegranate seeds.

In a small bowl, mix together the olive oil and balsamic vinegar and season with salt and pepper. Drizzle the dressing over the salad and serve.

Serves 1

1 little gem lettuce
½ cucumber, sliced
10–15 baby tomatoes in different colours, quartered
½ red onion, sliced
30g (1oz) feta, crumbled
handful of parsley, chopped
handful of pomegranate seeds
1 tbsp olive oil
1 tsp balsamic vinegar
sea salt and freshly ground black pepper

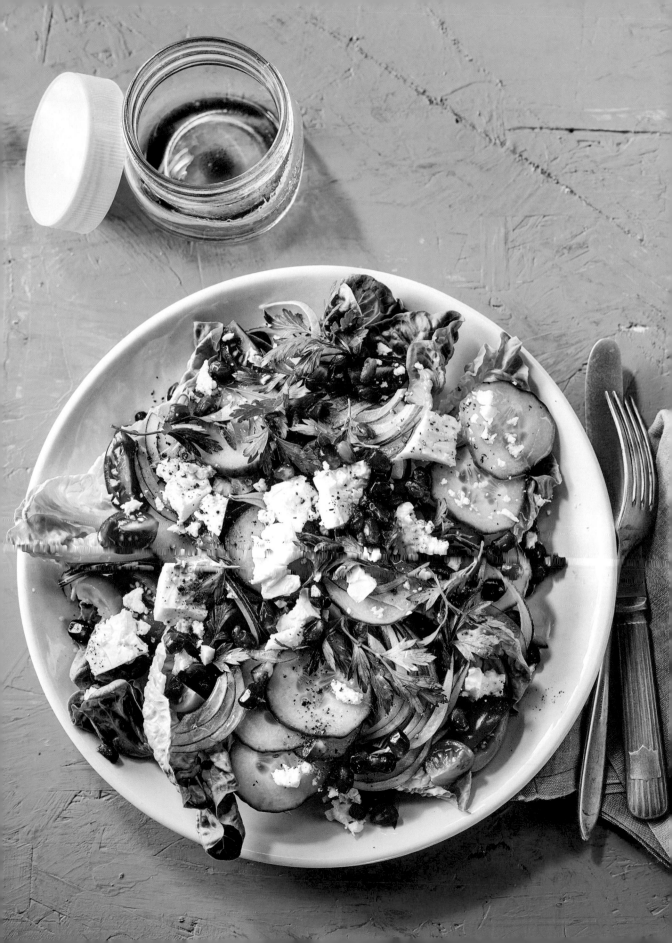

ULTRA-EASY SHAKSHUKA

This one-pan winner gets all its flavour from a small amount of chorizo. It's bold and feels like a real treat, but it's still healthy and easy to make as the eggs just poach themselves within the mixture.

Add the olive oil to a frying pan over a medium heat. When hot, add the onion and romano pepper and fry for 5–6 minutes until caramelized and soft. Add the chorizo and fry for a further 3–4 minutes.

Add the tomatoes to the pan and season with salt and pepper. Give everything a good stir and allow to simmer for 10 minutes.

Create two wells in the sauce with a spoon and crack an egg into each well.

Cover the pan with a lid and cook for 5–10 minutes, to your preference (10 minutes if you want eggs cooked all the way through).

Garnish with the parsley and serve.

Serves 2

1 tbsp olive oil
½ onion, sliced
1 romano pepper, deseeded and sliced
50g (1¾oz) chorizo, diced
½ x 400g (14oz) can chopped tomatoes
2 eggs
sea salt and freshly ground black pepper
1 tbsp chopped fresh parsley, to garnish

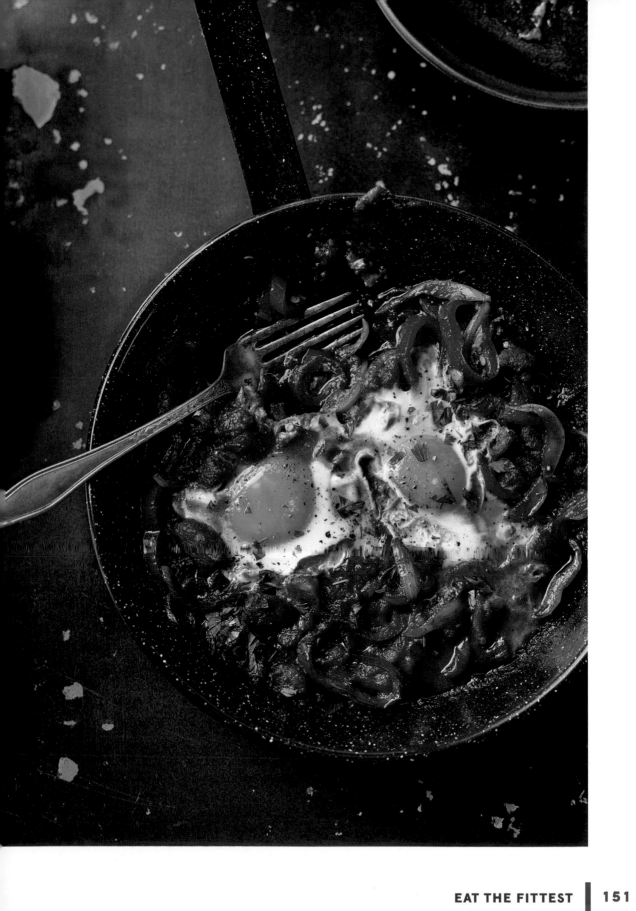

TY'S NOTHING-IN-THE-FRIDGE TASTY TUNA FOR TWO

Look at this! You just need to pick up olives and spinach on the way home and you probably already have the other ingredients in your kitchen cupboards. Then you can bang it out with no effort. This is high-protein gold after a bout of high-intensity training.

Heat the olive oil in a frying pan over a medium heat and when hot, add the onion. Fry for about 5–6 minutes until softened.

Add the garlic to the pan and cook for 2–3 minutes.

Add the tuna to the pan with the chopped tomatoes, olives and spinach and give everything a good stir to allow the spinach to wilt.

Add the vegetable stock, stir and simmer over a medium heat for 5–7 minutes until the sauce has reduced.

When the sauce begins to thicken, make 2 indents in the mixture with a spoon and crack the eggs into the indents. Cover and cook for a further 10–15 minutes over a medium heat until the eggs are cooked thoroughly.

Season with salt and pepper and drizzle the honey over. Serve.

Serves 2

1 tbsp olive oil
1 red onion, finely chopped
2 garlic cloves, crushed
2 x 145g (5oz) cans tuna, drained
1 x 400g (14oz) can chopped tomatoes
handful of mixed olives
200g (7oz) baby leaf spinach
285ml (1¼ cups) vegetable stock
2 eggs
1 tbsp honey
sea salt and freshly ground black pepper

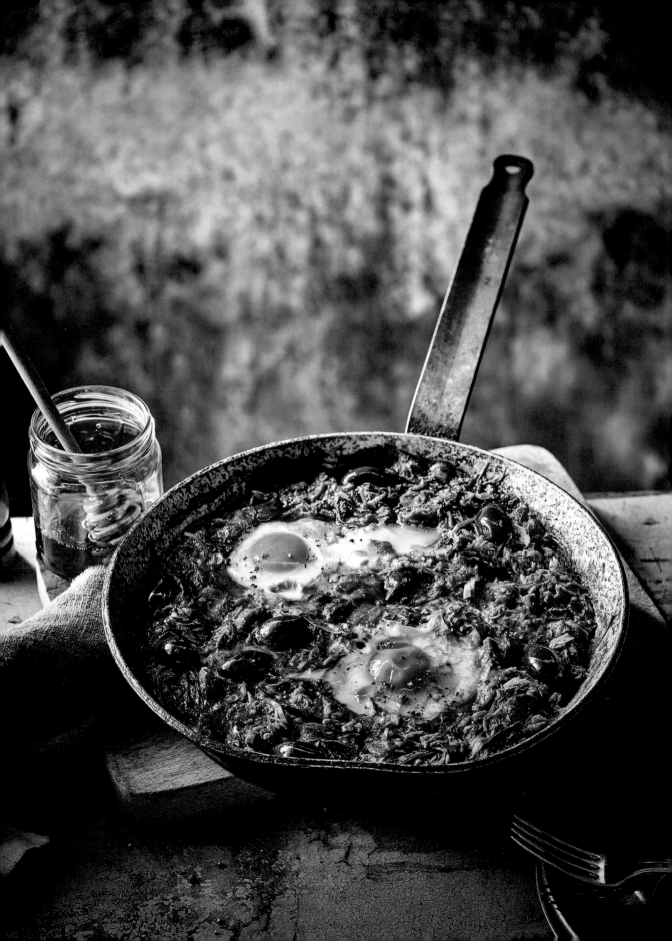

SIRLOIN STEAK & ROASTED TOMATO SALAD

When you want to treat yourself, this should be your go-to. Steak is rich and decadent but once in a while it's so good for you thanks to the iron, especially with the tomato salad. I don't often eat red meat but this is my precious exception!

Preheat the oven to 200°C/400°F/gas mark 6.

Put the tomatoes into a small roasting pan. Drizzle with a little olive oil followed by the soy sauce. Roast for 12 minutes, shaking the pan midway.

Heat a frying pan over a high heat. Lightly brush the sirloin steak with olive oil and season with salt and pepper to taste. When the pan is hot, add the steak and cook for 3–4 minutes each side for medium. Cook to your own preference, remove from the pan, reserving any juices in the pan, and set aside to rest for 3–4 minutes. Slice the steak.

Remove the tomatoes from the oven, reserving any juices in the pan.

Place the rocket (arugula) on a plate and drizzle with the balsamic vinegar. Top with the roasted tomatoes and sliced steak. Drizzle over any leftover cooking juices from the steak and tomatoes.

Serves 1

160g (5½oz) cherry tomatoes
1 tbsp olive oil
4 tbsp soy sauce
170g (6oz) sirloin steak
80g (3oz) rocket (arugula)
1 tsp balsamic vinegar
sea salt and freshly ground black pepper

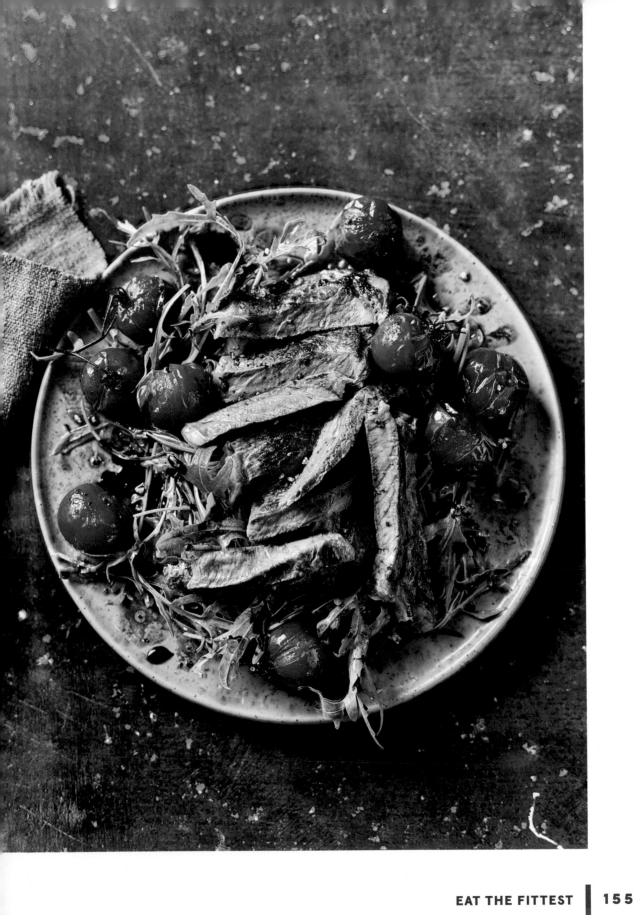

HEALTHIER HIGH-PROTEIN CHICKEN CAESAR SALAD

Everyone loves Caesar salad, right? But the dressing can be pretty calorific from the mayo. My version uses tofu that's blended to make a creamy dressing. You can make this salad for friends when you want to impress, knowing that it's healthier but still awesome.

Preheat the oven to 180°C/350°F/gas mark 4.

Bring a small pan of salted water to the boil and add the chicken leg. Simmer gently for 15–20 minutes. Remove the pan from the heat, but leave the chicken to cool in the water for 10 minutes.

Make the dressing. Add the tofu, anchovies, Parmesan and half the garlic clove to a food processor. Squeeze in a little lemon juice and blend until smooth. Set aside.

Rub the other half of the garlic clove over both sides of the sourdough bread. Place directly on an oven shelf and bake until toasted and crisp – about 5–7 minutes.

Bring a small pan of water to the boil, add the egg and simmer for 7 minutes. Remove from the water and hold under cold running water. Peel the egg and cut it in half.

Remove the chicken from the water. Pull the flesh (and skin, if using) from the bone and tear it into pieces. Discard the bone.

Take the sourdough out of the oven and cut it into small squares.

To assemble, put the lettuce, chicken, croutons and halved egg on a plate. Drizzle over the dressing, add pepper, and serve.

Serves 1

1 chicken leg, skin on or skinless as preferred
150g (5¼oz) silken tofu, cubed
4 anchovies
20g (¾oz) grated Parmesan
1 garlic clove
1 lemon
1 slice of sourdough bread
1 egg
1 Cos lettuce, torn into pieces
sea salt and freshly ground black pepper

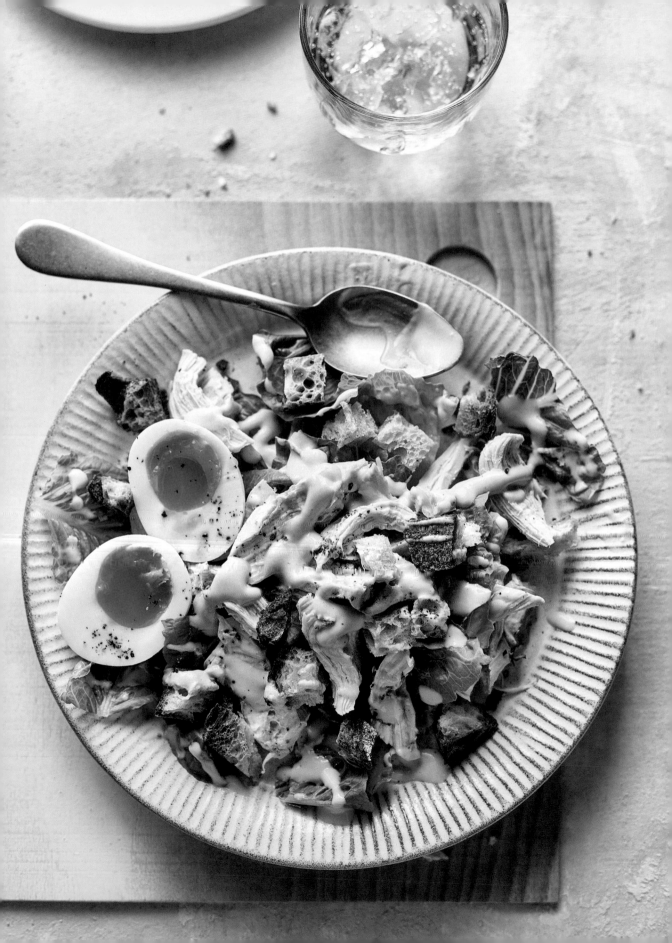

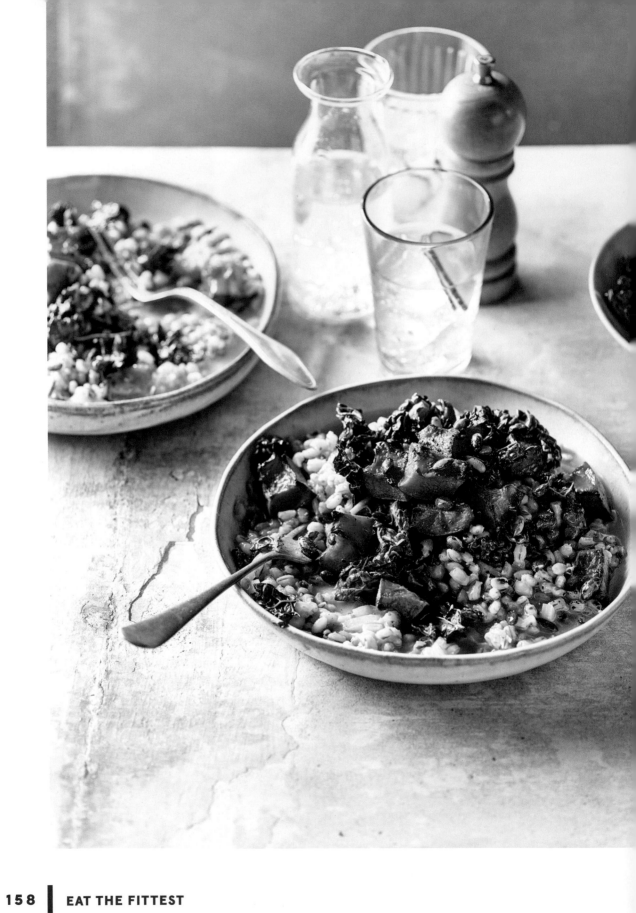

PEARL BARLEY RISOTTO WITH ROAST PUMPKIN

Pumpkin, high in antioxidants, helps with immunity and pearl barley is a nutritious alternative to white risotto rice and more satisfying. If you're vegetarian, try to find a Parmesan made without rennet, or substitute for a vegetarian equivalent.

Preheat the oven to 180°C/350°F/gas mark 4.

Place the pumpkin on a baking tray. Drizzle with olive oil and add a sprinkle of salt. Roast in the oven for 15–20 minutes until tender.

Toast the pearl barley in a dry pan over a medium heat until golden – about 5 minutes. Transfer the barley to a bowl and in the same pan, add half the olive oil to heat. Add the onion and barley again and cook gently for 5 minutes. You don't want the onion to start to colour.

Begin adding the vegetable stock – just enough to cover the barley – and a pinch of salt. As the liquid is absorbed by the barley, keep adding more stock until the barley is cooked and you have a thick risotto base.

Meanwhile, heat the remaining oil in a frying pan and sauté the cavolo nero or kale with the pumpkin seeds for 3–4 minutes.

Remove the risotto pan from the heat, stir through the Parmesan and finish with a squeeze of lemon. Check the seasoning.

Remove the pumpkin from the oven. Add the pumpkin seeds and greens and give it a stir, trying not to break up the pumpkin.

Place the risotto base in a bowl and top with the vegetables to serve.

Serves 2

150g (5¼oz) pumpkin, cut into 2cm (¾in) cubes
1 tbsp olive oil, plus extra for drizzling
100g (generous ½ cup) pearl barley
½ onion, finely diced
200ml (¾ cup) hot vegetable stock
50g (1¾oz) cavolo nero or kale, chopped
1 tbsp pumpkin seeds
20g (¾oz) Parmesan, finely grated
1 lemon
sea salt and freshly ground black pepper

BUTTERNUT SQUASH TAGINE WITH APRICOTS, PRUNES & QUINOA

Vg

Fruit in savoury dishes – if you've never tried it, do it now! There's loads of flavour from the dried apricots and prunes here and it just gets better the next day when the flavours have had time to develop.

Rinse the quinoa in cold water. Put 240ml (1 cup) water in a saucepan, add the quinoa and bring to the boil. Simmer for about 12 minutes or until all the water has evaporated and the quinoa has doubled in size, then remove from the heat.

Heat the olive oil in a pan over a low–medium heat and add the butternut squash. Cook gently for 15–20 minutes, allowing the pieces to caramelize slowly.

Add the apricots, prunes, cumin, paprika, ginger and garlic and sauté gently for a further 2 minutes.

Add the vegetable stock and simmer gently until all the stock has evaporated. Check the seasoning. Add a squeeze of lemon juice and a little salt.

Add the olives and stir through.

Serve alongside the quinoa with the coriander (cilantro) sprinkled over the top.

Serves 2

80g (scant ½ cup) quinoa
2 tbsp olive oil
200g (7oz) butternut squash, peeled and cut into 1cm (½in) cubes
20g (¾oz) chopped dried apricots
20g (¾oz) chopped prunes
10g (2 tsp) ground cumin
10g (2 tsp) paprika
5g (1 tsp) chopped fresh ginger
1 garlic clove, chopped
100ml (generous ⅓ cup) vegetable stock
1 lemon
15g (1 tbsp) chopped black olives
15g (1 tbsp) chopped fresh coriander (cilantro)
sea salt and freshly ground black pepper

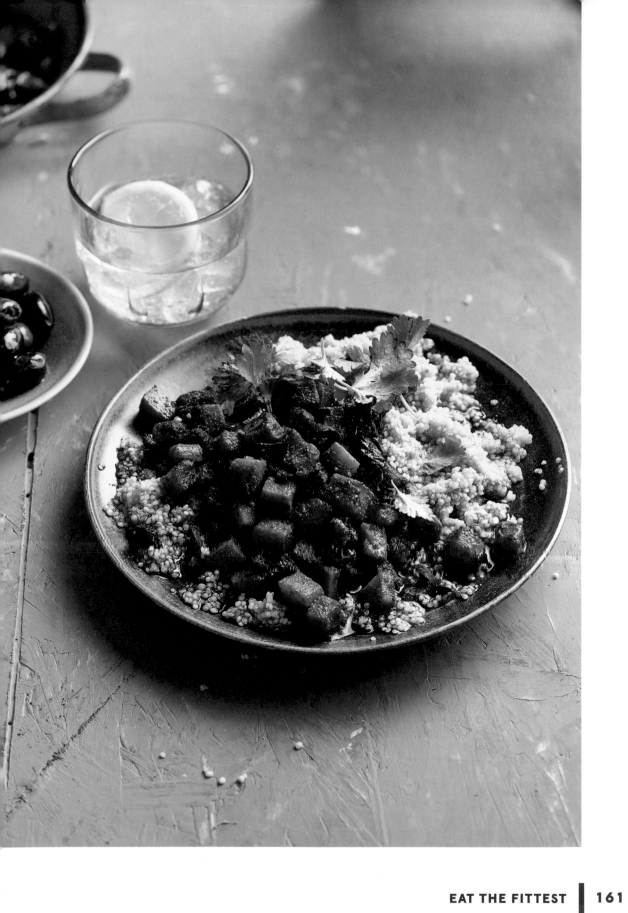

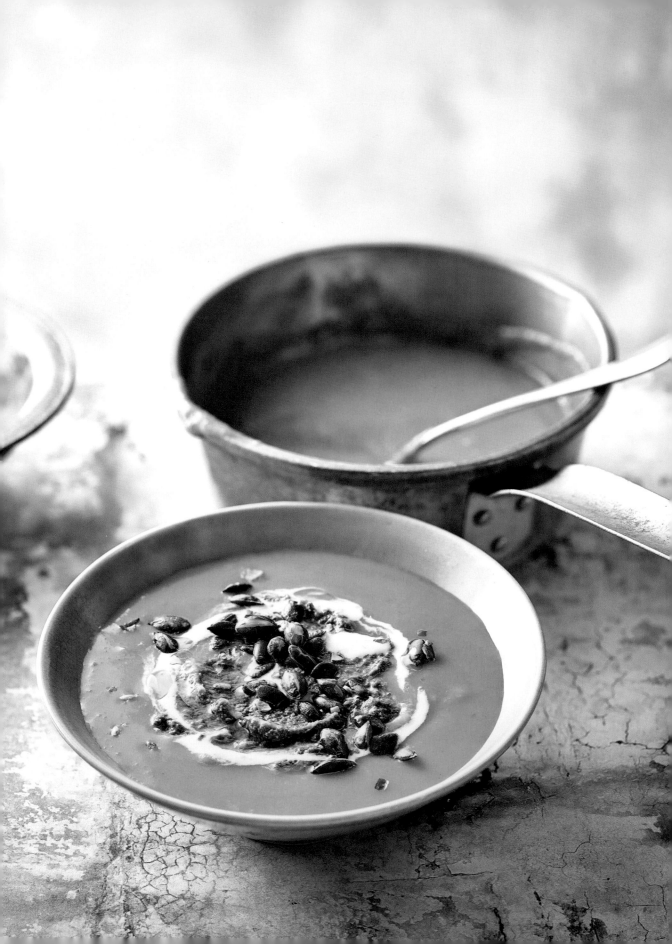

PUMPKIN SOUP WITH ROASTED PUMPKIN SEEDS & KALE PESTO

V

A good winter warmer of a soup, with a nutritious twist in the kale pesto on top. Pumpkin seeds are high in antioxidants, magnesium and fibre. If you're vegetarian, try to find a Parmesan made without rennet, or substitute for a vegetarian equivalent.

Preheat the oven to 180°C/350°F/gas mark 4.

Place the pumpkin on a baking tray, drizzle with a little olive oil and sprinkle with salt. Roast for 20 minutes until tender.

Add the kale to a food processor with half of the pumpkin seeds and all the Parmesan. Drizzle in a little olive oil and blend until smooth, adding more olive oil if needed. Season with salt and squeeze in a little lemon juice. Set aside.

Remove the pumpkin from the oven and transfer to a large saucepan. Add the vegetable stock, bring to the boil, then simmer for 10 minutes. Remove the pan from the heat, then blend until smooth using a food processor or stick blender.

Toast the remaining pumpkin seeds in a small, dry frying pan until they've puffed up a bit.

Put the soup into 2 serving bowls, drizzle the kale pesto over, then sprinkle the toasted pumpkin seeds on top. Finish with a tablespoon of yogurt and serve.

Serves 2

250g (9oz) pumpkin, peeled and cut into
  2cm (¾in) cubes
1–2 tbsp olive oil
100g (3½oz) kale
20g (¾oz) pumpkin seeds
10g (2 tsp) grated Parmesan
1 lemon
300ml (1¼ cups) vegetable stock
1 tbsp Greek yogurt or coconut yogurt

HOMEMADE LAMB KEBABS WITH THE WORKS

Swap that Friday late-night takeaway for this homemade version – just as good but much better for you and twice as satisfying because it's homemade!

First, make the kebabs. Place the lamb mince in a bowl and add the spices and garlic with a pinch of salt. Mix well, cover, place in the fridge and leave to marinate for 1 hour. Meanwhile leave 4 wooden kebab skewers to soak in water or use metal skewers instead.

Preheat the oven to 220°C/425°F/gas mark 7.

Remove the lamb from the fridge and divide the mixture into four equal portions. Mould each of the portions around a skewer so that you have four long, sausage-like shapes.

Place the kebabs on a baking tray and bake in the oven for 12–15 minutes, turning occasionally.

Put the yogurt into a small bowl with the mint and mix together.

Put the tomatoes and cucumber together in a bowl. Add the olive oil, balsamic vinegar and a pinch of salt and mix well to combine.

Remove the lamb from the oven and put the pittas into the oven to heat through for 1–2 minutes.

Pull the kebabs off the skewers onto a board and cut each one in half widthwise.

Take the pittas out of the oven and cut along the tops of one side to open them up.

Spoon the tomato and cucumber salad into the pittas, add the kebabs, then drizzle the mint yogurt inside.

Serves 2

200g (7oz) lamb mince
10g (2 tsp) ground cumin
5g (1 tsp) mild chilli powder
5g (1 tsp) paprika
2 garlic cloves, finely chopped
100g (3½oz) Greek yogurt
2 tbsp chopped fresh mint
2 tomatoes, finely diced
50g (1¾oz) cucumber, finely diced
2 tbsp olive oil
2 tsp balsamic vinegar
2 wholemeal pitta breads
salt

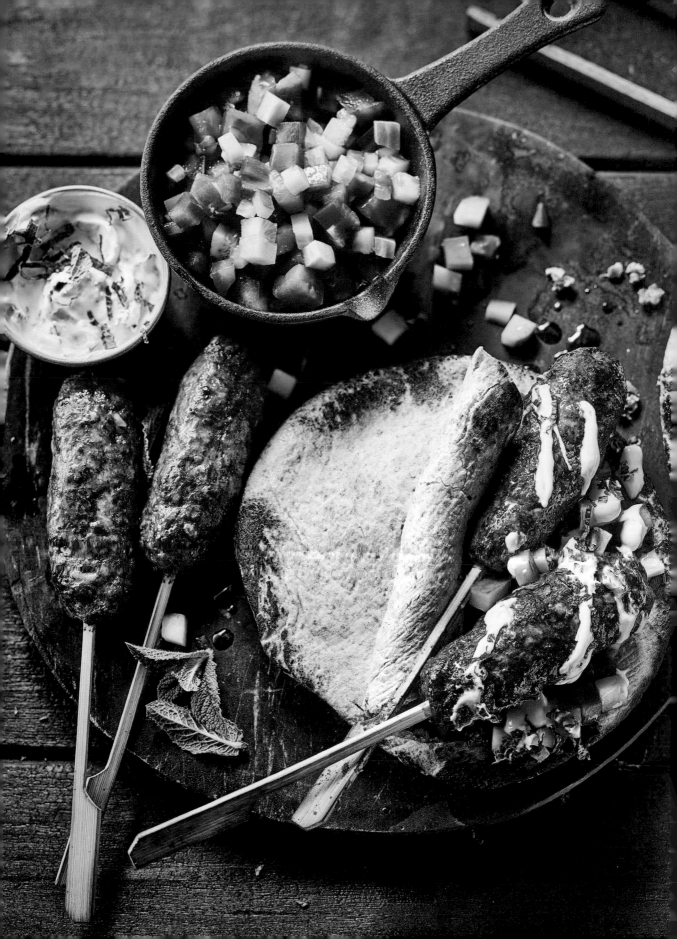

TANDOORI CHICKEN & CUCUMBER SALAD

Nothing is fried in this recipe but you'll be amazed how delicious it is. The yogurt helps to tenderize the chicken and the tandoori spice mix is an instant flavour bomb without any effort needed.

Preheat the oven to 220°C/425°F/gas mark 7. Line a baking tray with baking paper.

Mix the yogurt and the tandoori spice together in a small bowl.

Put the chicken pieces into a bowl and add half the yogurt mixture. Stir to coat all the pieces, then cover and put in the fridge to marinate for at least 10 minutes.

Add the mint and vinegar to the remaining tandoori yogurt. Set aside.

Remove the chicken from the marinade, place on the lined baking tray and bake in the oven for 15–20 minutes.

Using a vegetable peeler, peel the cucumber into ribbons.

Mix the lettuce and cucumber ribbons in a bowl and drizzle over the yogurt dressing.

Remove the chicken from the oven, place on top of the salad and serve.

Serves 1

50g (1¾oz) Greek yogurt
10g (2 tsp) tandoori spice mix
2 skinless, boneless chicken thighs, cut into
  5cm (2in) pieces
30g (2 tbsp) chopped fresh mint
1 tbsp white wine vinegar
½ cucumber
1 baby gem lettuce, sliced

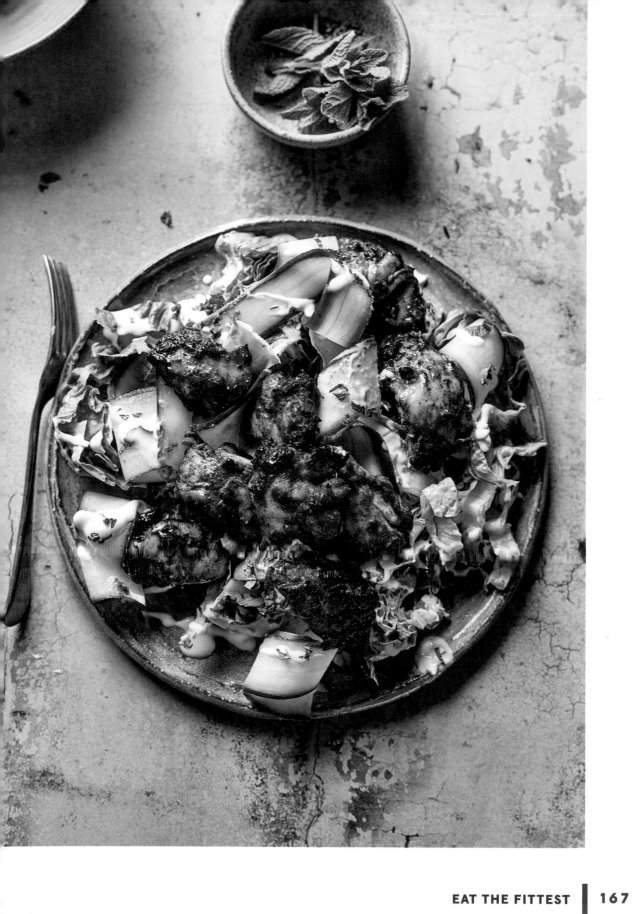

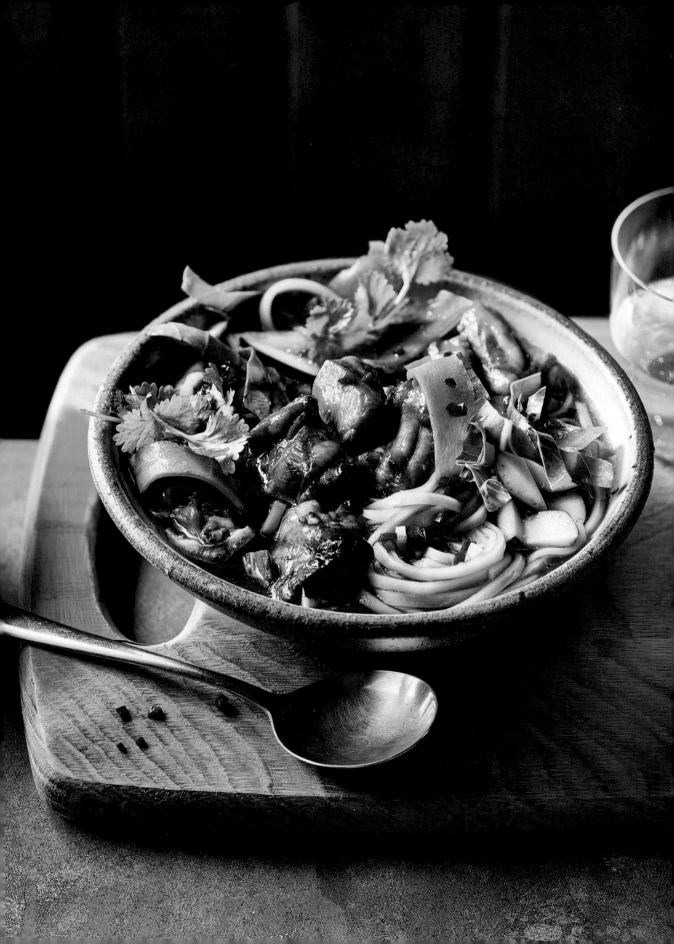

PUNCHY SOY & HONEY CHICKEN NOODLE SOUP WITH RAW VEG

Soy and honey together are a great combo – salty and sweet – and then when you cook them, you get a sweet, sticky sauce. This is a lovely dish packed with fresh veg, a punchy piece of chicken and fresh coriander to finish it all off.

Preheat the oven to 220°C/425°F/gas mark 7. Line a baking tray with baking paper.

Mix the soy sauce and honey together in a bowl and add the chicken pieces. Stir well to coat all the pieces. Cover and put into the fridge to marinate for at least 10 minutes.

Remove the chicken from the marinade and place on the lined baking tray. Bake in the oven for 15–20 minutes.

Pour the vegetable stock into a medium pan and bring to the boil. Add the miso and season with a little soy sauce.

Add the noodles and cook for 5 minutes.

Add the carrot, pak choi (bok choy) and courgette (zucchini) and remove the pan from the heat.

Remove the chicken from the oven and add it, with any cooking juices, to the broth.

Check the seasoning and adjust if necessary.

Ladle the broth into a serving bowl and sprinkle with the chilli and coriander (cilantro).

Serves 1

20ml (4 tsp) soy sauce
10ml (2 tsp) honey
2 skinless, boneless chicken thighs,
  cut into 2.5cm (1in) pieces
200ml (¾ cup) vegetable stock
2 tsp miso paste
1–2 tsp soy sauce
50g (1¾oz) rice noodles
1 carrot, peeled into ribbons
1 pak choi (bok choy), sliced
1 courgette (zucchini), thinly sliced
½ red chilli, finely chopped
50g (1¾oz) fresh coriander (cilantro)

FAST FISH SUPPER WITH COD, BROCCOLI, & SUN-DRIED TOMATOES

This is another of those top recipes that need hardly any ingredients, just a couple of easy bits from the local supermarket. It's efficient and the cod tastes amazing and soft baked in the oven like this.

Preheat the oven to 160°C/325°F/gas mark 3. Line a baking tray with baking paper.

Place the cod on the lined tray. Drizzle with 1 tsp of the olive oil and season with salt. Place in the oven and cook for 12–14 minutes.

Add the remaining olive oil to a frying pan over a medium heat. When hot, add the broccoli and allow to char on one side, about 6 minutes. Turn over, add the almonds and toast them with the broccoli for 6 minutes.

Cut the lemon in half and squeeze one half into the pan and season with salt.

Remove from the heat and add the sun-dried tomatoes. Toss through the broccoli.

Remove the cod from the oven and place the cod on a serving plate. Add the broccoli and sun-dried tomatoes alongside.

Drizzle with another squeeze of lemon juice and serve.

Serves 1

150g (5¼oz) skinless cod fillet
1 tbsp olive oil
200g (7oz) Tenderstem broccoli
2 tsp flaked (slivered) almonds
1 lemon
50g (1¾oz) sun-dried tomatoes, chopped
sea salt

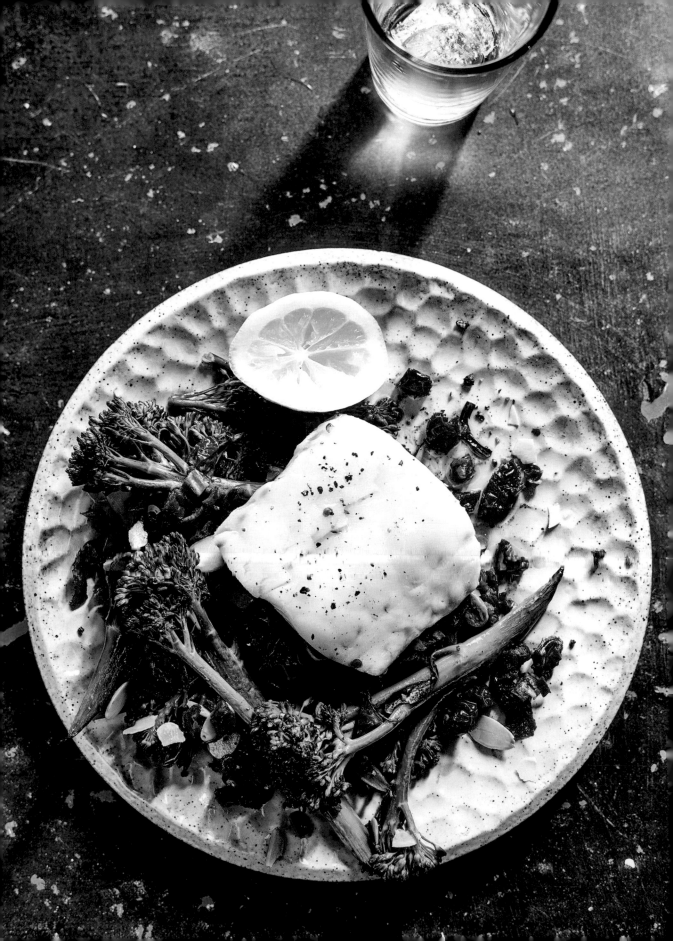

MISO- & SOY- MARINATED COD WITH BROWN RICE & PAK CHOI

This is bound to become a weeknight favourite as it ticks all the boxes: depth of flavour, nutrition and satisfaction. The cod keeps it light but miso, honey and soy sauce add a kick, the salad is fresh, and the peanuts give a great texture. This dish has it all!

Mix the miso, vinegar, honey and soy sauce together in a bowl for the marinade. Set 2 tbsp aside for dressing the salad.

Place the cod in the bowl with the marinade, making sure it's fully coated. Leave to stand for 15 minutes.

Preheat the oven to 220°C/425°F/gas mark 7. Line a baking tray with baking paper.

Remove the cod from the marinade and place on the lined baking tray. Spoon over any marinade that's left in the bowl, place in the oven and cook for 15 minutes.

Cook the rice according to the packet instructions.

Make the dressing. Add the spring onion (scallion), chilli, peanuts and pak choi (bok choy) to a bowl, pour over the reserved marinade and mix well.

Drain the rice and remove the cod from the oven. Put the rice into a serving bowl, place the cod on top and spoon over the dressing.

Serves 1

2–3 tbsp miso paste
1 tbsp rice vinegar
1 tbsp honey
1 tbsp soy sauce
150g (5¼oz) cod fillet
50g (¼ cup) brown rice
1 spring onion (scallion), finely sliced
1 red chilli, finely chopped
1 tbsp crushed roasted peanuts
1 pak choi (bok choy), sliced

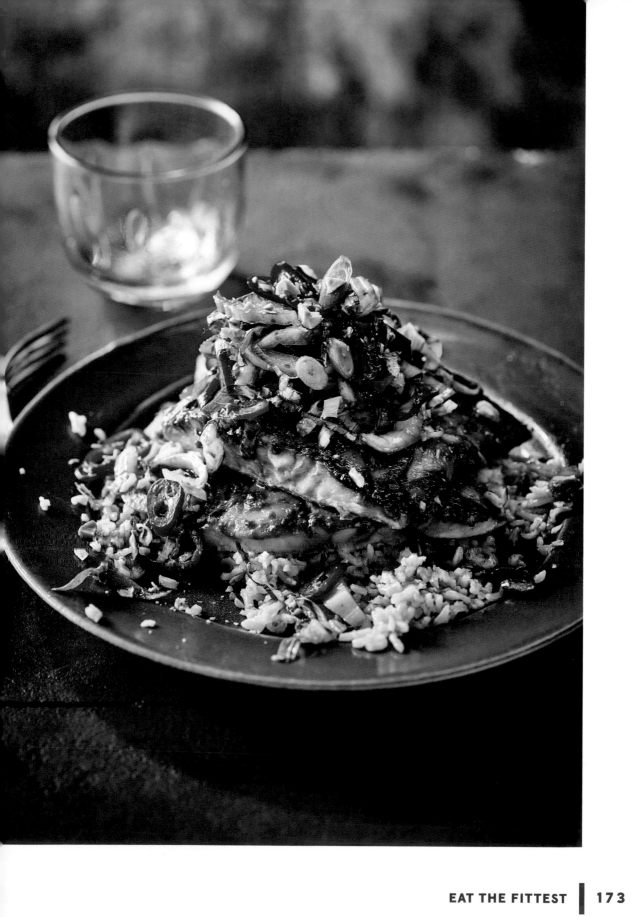

SNACKS

Vg
BLACK BEAN HUMMUS

Chickpeas and black beans with chilli flakes make for an amazing dip with raw veg sticks.

Serves 2

½ x 400g (14oz) can black beans, drained and rinsed
½ x 400g (14oz) can chickpeas (garbanzo beans), drained and rinsed
2–3 garlic cloves, to taste
juice of 1 lime
2 tbsp chopped fresh coriander (cilantro)
¼ tsp dried chilli flakes
½ tsp ground cumin
2 tbsp tahini
2 tbsp olive oil, plus extra for drizzling
sea salt and freshly ground black pepper

To serve
1 cucumber, cut into batons
2 carrots, cut into batons

Put the black beans and chickpeas (garbanzo beans) into a food processor and add the garlic, lime juice, coriander (cilantro), chilli flakes, cumin and tahini.

Whiz together until smooth and thick. With the food processor running gently, gradually add the olive oil and season to taste.

Transfer to a small bowl and drizzle with a little extra oil. Serve with the cucumber and carrot batons.

Vg
AVOCADO DIP WITH CHILLI & LIME

Use non-dairy yogurt if you want this to be vegan. It's a nice riff on guacamole.

Serves 2

2 avocados, peeled and stoned
handful of fresh parsley
handful of fresh coriander (cilantro)
3 tbsp lime juice
1 red chilli, chopped and deseeded
2 tbsp Greek yogurt or non-dairy yogurt
sea salt and freshly ground black pepper

To serve
3 carrots, cut into batons
handful of raw cauliflower florets

Put the avocados, herbs, lime juice, chilli and yogurt into a food processor. Blend until smooth and season to taste.

Transfer to a small bowl and serve with the carrots and cauliflower florets.

ROASTED BEETROOT FRIES WITH TANDOORI YOGURT

Potato fries can step aside – these beetroot fries are going to change your life! Use non-dairy yogurt if you want this to be vegan.

Preheat the oven to 200°C/400°F/gas mark 6. Line a baking sheet with baking paper.

Spread the beetroot (beet) fries over the baking sheet in a single layer and brush the olive oil over them. Place the beetroot in the oven for 20 minutes, turning halfway through cooking. It should be soft when you insert a sharp knife into one of the fries.

Put the yogurt into a small bowl, add all the spices and mix. Season generously.

Remove the fries from the oven, transfer to a serving bowl and serve with the tandoori spiced yogurt, sprinkled with the parsley.

Serves 2

2 beetroot (beets), peeled and cut into 5mm (¼in) fries
½ tbsp olive oil
5 tbsp plain yogurt or non-dairy yogurt
½ tsp ground coriander
½ tsp ground cumin
½ tsp ground turmeric
½ tsp cayenne pepper
½ tsp garam masala
½ tsp paprika
sea salt and freshly ground black pepper
chopped parsley, to serve

BAKED, SPICED APPLE CHIPS

Make these once and you'll realize how addictive they are!

Preheat the oven to 90°C/200°F/gas mark ¼. Line two baking sheets with baking paper.

Arrange the apple slices on the lined baking sheets in a single layer and sprinkle with half of the cinnamon and mixed spice.

Place both trays in the oven for 45 minutes. Remove from the oven, turn all the apple slices over and sprinkle with the remaining spices. Return to the oven for a further 45 minutes. They should look dried out by the end of cooking.

Remove from the oven and allow to cool completely. Serve with almond butter to spread on the slices, if you like. Store in an airtight container and eat within 2 days.

Serves 2

3 large Granny Smith apples, cored and
  thinly sliced
1 tsp ground cinnamon
1 teaspoon mixed spice
almond butter, to serve (optional)

BE THE FITTEST SMOOTHIE

Vg

This has got some serious oomph for those times when you need a quick, sharp pick-me-up.

Add all the ingredients to a food processor and blend thoroughly until smooth.

Serves 1

250ml (1 generous cup) coconut milk
30g (2 tbsp) almond butter
1 tsp pea protein powder
1 tsp hemp protein powder
140g (¾ cup) frozen blueberries
½ banana
1 tsp açaí powder
1 drop of vanilla extract

SAMPLE DIET PLANS

Here is an example of the diet on a three-week planner. Feel free to change the recipes around as much as you want for your own plan – make it your own. However, please stick to The Rules (page 77) and the schedule that I have suggested.

The snacks are optional, and are in case you are feeling hungry.

If eating breakfast as early as 7:30am doesn't suit you, or you don't feel like eating a meal first thing in the morning, swap around the 7:30am breakfast meals with the 10am optional snacks, or choose one or the other.

Try to plan out your meals like this every week. It will make grocery shopping easier, and if you know what you're having every day, it will mean that you won't be tempted to go for less healthy options.

1	7:30AM Breakfast	10AM Optional snack	1PM Lunch	4PM Optional snack	7PM Dinner
MONDAY	Bircher muesli (page 84)	The orange one (page 82)	Roast chicken, pepper & courgette salad (page 101)	Black bean hummus (page 174)	Super-easy, super-fresh baked salmon parcels (page 146)
TUESDAY	The green one (page 82)	Avocado dip with chilli & lime (page 174)	Blackened salmon with sweet potato, carrot & broccoli mash (page 123)	The vitamin one (page 83)	Pumpkin soup with roasted pumpkin seeds & kale pesto (page 163)
WEDNESDAY	Ty's killer avocado toast with mojo verde & poached egg (page 86)	The red one (page 82)	The king of salads, with garlic king prawns (page 102)	Baked, spiced apple chips (page 176)	Be the Fittest Mediterranean salad (page 148)
THURSDAY	Porridge with berries (page 84)	The energy one (page 83)	Miso-roasted cauliflower with kale pesto & cherry tomatoes (page 116)	Roasted beetroot fries with tandoori yogurt (page 175)	Butternut squash tagine with apricots, prunes & quinoa (page 160)
FRIDAY	The best breakfast omelette (page 88)	Avocado dip with chilli & lime (page 174)	Jerusalem artichoke soup with poached eggs & sautéed mushrooms (page 110)	The post-workout one (page 83)	Sirloin steak & roasted tomato salad (page 154)
SATURDAY	Healthy veggie English breakfast (page 93)	The on-the-go one (page 83)	Spiced marinated cod with noodle broth & raw veg (page 115)	Be the Fittest smoothie (page 177)	Homemade lamb kebabs with the works (page 164)
SUNDAY	Smoked salmon & chilli avocado with poached egg on toast (page 94)	The green one (page 82)	Fit fish pie with broccoli & mangetout (page 97)	Roasted beetroot fries with tandoori yogurt (page 175)	Miso- and soy-marinated cod with brown rice & pak choi (page 172)

2	7:30AM Breakfast	10AM Optional snack	1PM Lunch	4PM Optional snack	7PM Dinner
MONDAY	Mighty greens on sourdough toast (page 93)	The energy one (page 83)	Baked sweet potato with tuna, chilli & lime (page 124)	Avocado dip with chilli & lime (page 174)	Tandoori chicken & cucumber salad (page 166)
TUESDAY	Coconut yogurt bowl (page 85)	The red one (page 82)	Steamed hake with green lentil dhal & kale (page 113)	The post-workout one (page 83)	Fast fish supper with cod, broccoli & sun-dried tomatoes (page 170)
WEDNESDAY	Granola with fruit & seeds (page 85)	The orange one (page 82)	Baked paprika chicken with brown rice (page 120)	Roasted beetroot fries with tandoori yogurt (page 175)	Punchy soy & honey chicken noodle soup with raw veg (page 169)
THURSDAY	Smoked salmon & chilli avocado with poached egg on toast (page 94)	The red one (page 82)	Aubergine & tofu curry with brown rice (page 126)	Black bean hummus (page 174)	Ultra-easy shakshuka (page 150)
FRIDAY	The best breakfast omelette (page 88)	The energy one (page 83)	Mackerel, tomato & red onion rice salad (page 130)	Be the Fittest smoothie (page 177)	Sirloin steak & roasted tomato salad (page 154)
SATURDAY	The vitamin one (page 83)	Post-workout açaí bowl (page 92)	Spinach, tofu, chickpea & potato curry (page 132)	Baked, spiced apple chips (page 176)	The ultimate chicken salad (page 142)
SUNDAY	Healthy veggie English breakfast (page 93)	The on-the-go one (page 83)	Vegan full-of-beans burger (page 129)	Baked, spiced apple chips (page 176)	Pearl barley risotto with roast pumpkin (page 159)

3	**7:30AM** Breakfast	**10AM** Optional snack	**1PM** Lunch	**4PM** Optional snack	**7PM** Dinner
MONDAY	Ty's killer avocado toast with mojo verde & poached egg (page 86)	The green one (page 82)	Heritage tomato salad with caramelized peaches, mozzarella & olives (page 107)	Black bean hummus (page 174)	The ultimate chicken salad (page 142)
TUESDAY	Coconut yogurt bowl (page 85)	The green one (page 82)	Jerusalem artichoke soup with poached eggs & sautéed mushrooms (page 110)	Roasted beetroot fries with tandoori yogurt (page 175)	Be The Fittest mediterranean salad (page 148)
WEDNESDAY	Porridge with berries (page 84)	Black bean hummus (page 174)	Roast chicken, pepper & courgette salad (page 101)	Baked, spiced apple chips (page 176)	Superfood salad with quinoa, tofu, beetroot, & aubergine (page 139)
THURSDAY	Scrambled eggs with smoked salmon (page 89)	The energy one (page 83)	Couscous with peppers, broccoli, capers, pine nuts & almonds (page 118)	Avocado dip with chilli & lime (page 174)	Rice bowl with brown rice, tofu, greens & a poached egg (page 143)
FRIDAY	Bircher muesli (page 84)	The green one (page 82)	Spiced marinated cod with noodle broth & raw veg (page 115)	Be the Fittest smoothie (page 177)	Tandoori chicken & cucumber salad (page 166)
SATURDAY	Granola with fruit & seeds (page 85)	The red one (page 82)	Fit fish pie with broccoli & mangetout (page 97)	Avocado dip with chilli & lime (page 174)	Butternut squash tagine with apricots, prunes & quinoa (page 160)
SUNDAY	Coconut yogurt bowl (page 85)	Baked, spiced apple chips (page 176)	Healthier roast chicken & potatoes with cabbage & carrots (page 135)	The orange one (page 82)	Punchy soy & honey chicken noodle soup with raw veg (page 169)

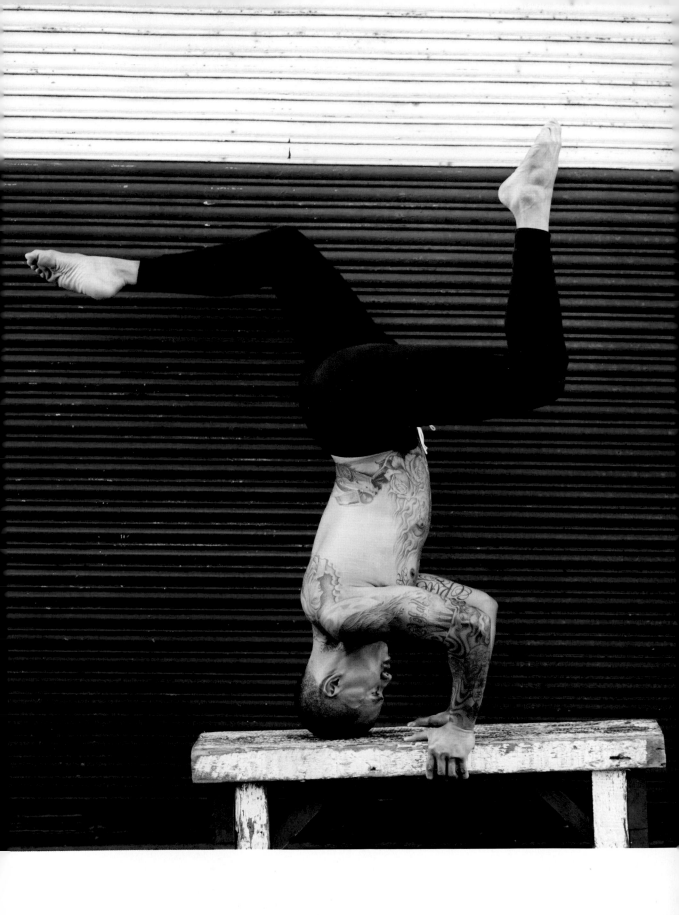

2A

3

FEEL
THE
FITTEST

This chapter is all about your mind. You will learn how to explore your inner feelings, going deeper within yourself to discover how to help yourself feel better through yoga, meditation and breathing. This practice should go hand in hand with your training programme.

I have trained from a young age, but a lot of my sports and fitness consisted of weights and cardio, so I found that I lacked a lot of flexibility and mobility. I was never really taught how to stretch properly. I was so stiff that I couldn't even touch my toes without bending my legs, I had a really tight neck and I had a lot of issues with my shoulders, to the point that I dislocated a shoulder in 2010.

In 2015 I was training one of my male clients to help him get ready for the Olympics. I explained to him that he needed to improve his flexibility and that one way to do that (I had heard) was to go to yoga classes. He initially refused, and said that the only way he would go to yoga was if I came with him. So we started going to yoga classes together! To be honest, at first I found it pretty tough, but it was here that my yoga journey began.

When I first started doing yoga, the aim (for myself and my client) was purely to become more flexible and mobile. I wanted it to act as a support to my training and overall fitness. As I started to practise more frequently, I learnt more about it as a discipline and was able to progress with the breathing exercises, as well as the spiritual side of the practice, along with seated meditation.

I now believe very passionately that we should all look at integrating a lifestyle of exercise and fitness with yoga and meditation. I see yoga as a discipline, but also as a tool for life which helps keep the body physically mobile, strong and supple but also teaches us how to breathe. This allows us to relax and stay calm through difficult situations in life as they occur, and gives us the tools to stay mentally stable and experience a better overall feeling of wellbeing. Exercise alone doesn't always allow us to achieve this.

The yoga that I learnt when I first started was ashtanga yoga. I learnt the foundations and then practised a lot more different styles. Throughout the years of practising yoga I have experimented, and have taken the bits from each style of yoga asana (poses) that I feel are most important to help someone that comes from a fitness and sports background, in order to create the most efficient practice for them.

What is yoga?

When I first tried yoga I didn't understand at all what it was or what I was doing; I just thought of it as a class where people went and stretched for an hour. I soon realized that yoga is much deeper and more spiritual than this.

The word 'yoga' comes from the Sanskrit root 'yuj', which means 'to yoke, attach or form a union'. There are many ways that yoga can be interpreted but for me it is a tool that allows you to bring the physical and internal self together as one, or to withdraw your mind from external activities.

What is meditation?

Meditation has been used in religions like Hinduism and Buddhism for centuries to reach a path of enlightenment. It is spiritual, but it is also invaluable for people who suffer from anxieties or fear; for when your brain feels jumbled. It helps to create mental clarity. This is scientifically proven as are its physical benefits, such as aiding in lowering blood pressure. Meditation enables you to stay calm and in control and to make good decisions. That's why I use meditation like a tool for life. For anyone who hasn't tried it before, think of it as awareness of your internal and external self.

Why is wellbeing important?

I'm a firm believer in balance. When exercising, you push the body and mind to their limits, so you need to know how to relax them, too. You need balance. You shouldn't overload the body and you should always remember to look after yourself.

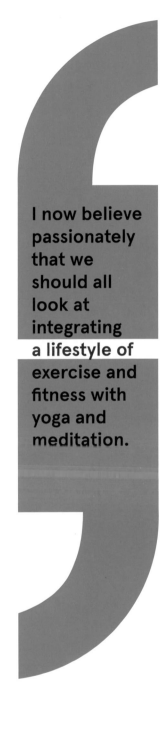

I now believe passionately that we should all look at integrating a lifestyle of exercise and fitness with yoga and meditation.

There are many types of yoga, but this yoga derives from ashtanga yoga. Every Yoga Practice starts with a warm-up in the form of Sun Salutations A and B. Then you'll do a number of poses and finish with the cool-down Padmasana and Savasana. Choose the right level as required in the 12-week programme (pages 68–73).

When you do a yoga pose, every movement has a breath – an inhale and an exhale. When you first try a pose, take your time and do each step. Try to remember what you're doing, then the next time you do it, you will know what's coming next. Over time I want you to memorize these poses and do them from memory.

You must use your ujjayi breath along with your bandhas.

Ujjayi breath: victorious breath

This is a controlled long and smooth breathing in and out of the nose. During your practice, try to restrict the opening of the throat passage which will allow you to be able to breathe more slowly and create a slow soothing sound, often sounding like an ocean. The quantity of the inhalation and exhalation are equal.

Bandhas: internal locks

These bandhas are internal locks which you should implement from the start to the end of the practice. There are two main locks I want you to concentrate on and engage.

Mula bandha: the toning and control of the pelvic floor muscle is responsible for providing the root foundation. This involves slightly squeezing your perineum throughout the practice.

Udiyana bandha: This is the toning and drawing in of the lower abdomen and

provides the result of upward flying energy. This is a contracting of your abdomen towards your spine.

The yoga practice

Beginner
· 3 x Sun Salutation A *(page 188)*
· 2 x Sun Salutation B *(pages 189–191)*
· The 5 yoga poses from page 192 to 196
· Finish with Padmasana *(page 207)* and Savasana *(page 208)*

Intermediate
· 3 x Sun Salutation A *(page 188)*
· 3 x Sun Salutation B *(pages 189–191)*
· The 11 poses from page 192 to 202
· Finish with Padmasana *(page 207)* and Savasana *(page 208)*

Advanced
· 5 x Sun Salutation A *(page 188)*
· 5 x Sun Salutation B *(pages 189–191)*
· The poses from page 192 to 206
· Finish with Padmasana *(page 207)* and Savasana *(page 208)*

Opposite are some of the basic poses you'll find mentioned regularly in yoga.

Words of encouragement

If you've never done yoga before, don't worry. Before I first tried it, I didn't really know what it was and I didn't understand what it could do for me. Initially I did it to become stronger and more flexible. Then I began to appreciate the mental benefits thanks to the breathing techniques and meditation. All of this combined is what makes yoga different from any other type of exercise.

Remember, keep practising. Even if you think you're not making progress, you are. I have been there, too; I used to doubt I could ever do some of the moves. Consistency is key; slow and steady. Don't let lack of flexibility discourage you. Over time you will open up.

Mountain pose

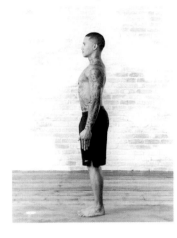

Prayer position

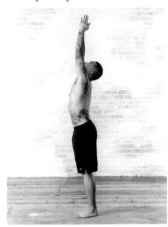

Downward facing dog

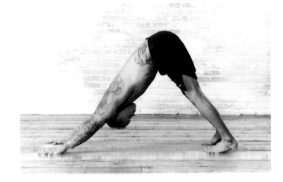

Chaturanga

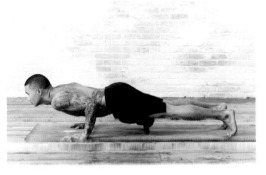

Warrior one

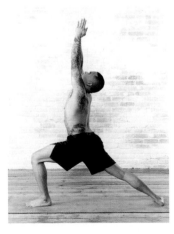

Upward facing dog

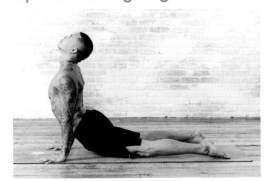

SUN SALUTATION A
SURYA NAMASKAR A

Repeat this sequence as requested in the programme, followed by Sun Salutation B.

1 Begin by standing in mountain pose.

2 Inhale as you bring your hands together over your head, hands in prayer position, keeping your arms straight, and look towards your hands.

3 Exhale, hands down to the floor and forward fold, place your hands flat beside your feet. Keep your legs bent if you lack flexibility in your hamstrings, or straighten your legs if you can, and bring your head towards your knees or shins.

4 Inhale, bring your head up, keeping your back straight.

5 Exhale, step or jump your feet back to plank pose, then straight into chaturanga.

6 Inhale, roll forward to your upward facing dog, opening your chest and bringing your shoulders away from your ears.

7 Exhale, tuck your toes under and go into a downward facing dog. Remain here for 5 long inhalations and exhalations.

8 On an inhale step or jump your feet between your hands.

9 Exhale, fold forward, bringing your head towards your knees.

10 Inhale, coming up to standing, bringing your hands over your head and looking towards your hands in prayer position.

11 Exhale, hands back down to your sides to standing.

SUN SALUTATION B
SURYA NAMASKAR B

Repeat this sequence as requested in the programme, after doing Sun Salutation A.

See pages 190–191 for photos.

1 Begin by standing in mountain pose.

2 Bend your knees. Inhale as you bring your hands together over your head, hands in prayer position, keeping your arms straight, and look towards your hands.

3 Exhale, hands down to the floor and forward fold, place your hands flat beside your feet. Keep your legs bent if you lack flexibility in your hamstrings, or straighten your legs if you can, and bring your head towards your knees or shins.

4 Inhale, bring your head up, keeping your back straight.

5 Exhale, step or jump your feet back to plank pose, then lower your body towards the floor keeping your elbows tucked into your sides, to chaturanga.

6 Inhale, roll forward to your upward facing dog, opening your chest and bringing your shoulders away from your ears.

7 Exhale, tuck your toes under and go into a downward facing dog.

8 Inhale, turn your left heel in, stepping your right foot between your hands and bringing your hands over your head, arms straight and hips square. Look towards your hands in warrior one.

9 Exhale, step your right leg back to plank pose, then into chaturanga.

10 Inhale, roll forward to your upward facing dog, opening your chest and bringing your shoulders away from your ears.

11 Exhale, tuck your toes under and go into a downward facing dog.

12 Bring your right heel in, stepping your left foot between your hands and bringing your hands over your head, arms straight and hips square. Look towards your hands in warrior one.

13 Exhale, step your left leg back to plank pose, then into chaturanga.

14 Inhale, roll forward to your upward facing dog, opening your chest and bringing your shoulders away from your ears.

15 Exhale, tuck your toes under and go into a downward facing dog. Remain here for 5 long inhalations and exhalations.

16 On an inhale step or jump your feet between your hands.

17 Exhale, fold forward, bringing your head towards your knees.

18 Inhale, coming up, keeping your legs bent and bringing your hands over your head. Look towards your hands in prayer position, keeping your back straight.

19 Exhale, hands back down to your sides to standing.

SUN SALUTATION B

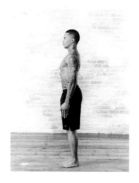 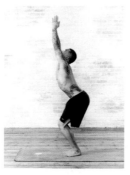 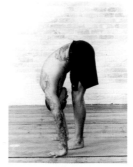 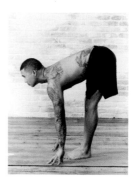

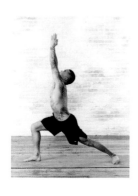 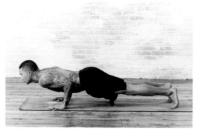 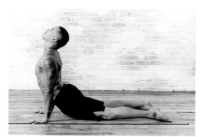

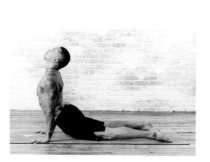 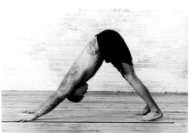 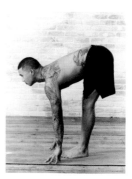

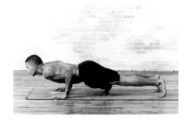
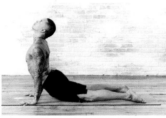
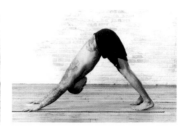

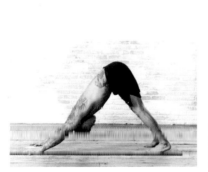
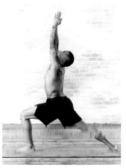
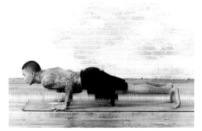

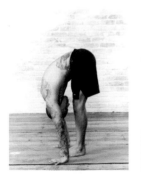
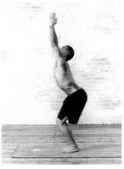
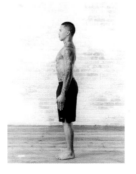

PADANGUSTHASANA
STANDING BIG TOE FOLD

Good for stretching your calves, hamstrings, hips and lower back. You may need a strap.

1 Begin in a standing position with your feet parallel, just less then hip width apart. Keeping your legs completely straight, exhale and bend forward, folding from your hip joints, keeping your back as straight as you can, moving your torso and head towards your shin and knees.

2 Slide the two forefingers and thumb of each hand between the big toe and second toe of each foot. Curl and wrap those fingers under and grip the big toes firmly, wrapping the thumbs around the other two fingers to secure the grip. Press your toes down against your fingers. If you struggle to reach your toes use a strap – place it under your feet and hold either side of your feet.

3 Inhale, raise your torso, lifting your head, creating space around your stomach. Straighten your elbows and back. Lengthen your torso, and on the next exhale, start to fold forward. As you do this, begin to straighten your hamstrings while pulling on the strap (if using).

4 Bend your elbows out to the sides and try to suck your belly in, lengthen the front and sides of your torso and through each breath gently lower more into the forward bend. If your hamstrings are flexible you can bring your forehead toward your shins. If your hamstrings are tight then focus on keeping your back in a safe position – as straight as you can – but at the same time feeling the stretch in your hamstrings.

5 Remain here for 5–10 long breaths. Then release the grip from your toes, bring your hands to your hips. Straighten your back and lift your head. With an inhale, come back up to standing.

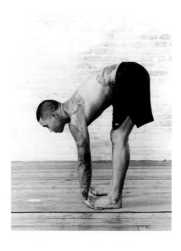
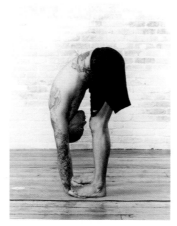

UTTHITA TRIKONASANA
TRIANGLE POSE

Good for stretching your hips, hamstrings and torso. You may need a block if you can't reach your hands to your ankles.

1 Begin in mountain pose.

2 On an exhalation, step your right foot out so that your feet are 90–120cm (3–4 feet) apart. Inhale, raise your arms up parallel to the floor and reach them out to the sides, keeping your arms straight and palms down.

3 Turn your left foot in slightly to the right so the foot is diagonal. Your right foot should be out, facing forwards and leading. Align the right heel with the left heel. Turn your right thigh outward, so that the right kneecap is in line with the centre of the right foot.

4 Exhale and extend the torso to the right. Bring your right arm down towards your right leg, bending from the hip joint and sucking your belly in.

5 Rest your right hand on your shin or ankle, or grab your big toe with your two forefingers and thumb, creating a wrap around the big toe. Stretch your left arm towards the ceiling. Keep your head in a neutral position or turn it to the left looking up towards the ceiling, you should be looking towards your left hand.

6 Stay in this pose for 5 long deep breaths. Inhale to come up, strongly pressing your feet to the floor and using your core. Reverse the feet and repeat these steps for the same length of time on the left side.

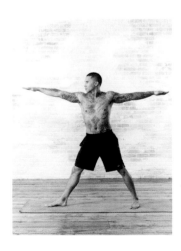
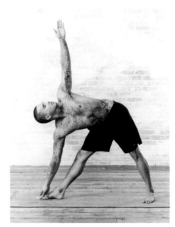

PARIVRTTA TRIKONASANA
REVOLVED TRIANGLE POSE

Good for stretching your hamstrings, calves, hips, torso and spine. You may need a block.

1 Begin in mountain pose.

2 On an exhalation, step your right foot out so that your feet are 90–120cm (3–4 feet) apart. Inhale, raise your arms up parallel to the floor and reach them out to the sides, keeping your arms straight and palms down.

3 Turn your left foot in slightly to the right so the foot is diagonal. Your right foot should be out, facing forwards and leading. Align the right heel with the left heel. Turn your right thigh outward, so that the right kneecap is in line with the centre of the right foot.

4 On an exhale, square your hips turning your torso to the right. Then twist your hips and start to bring your left hand down towards the floor to your right foot.

5 Reach your left hand down, either onto the floor outside the right foot or ankle, or, if you can't reach the floor, place your hand on a block. Keep twisting through your hips and keep your legs strong. Bring your right arm up in the air with your hand pointing towards the ceiling. If you have any neck issues keep your head in a neutral position, looking straight forward. Alternatively look up towards your right hand.

6 Stay in this pose for 5–10 long breaths. Exhale, release the twist and bring your torso back to upright with an inhalation to standing. Repeat the same steps on the other side.

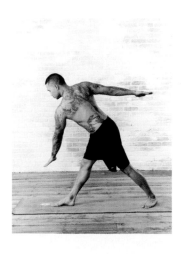 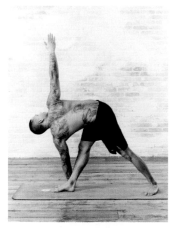

UTTHITA PARSVAKONASANA
EXTENDED SIDE ANGLE POSE

Good for stretching your spine, torso, hamstrings and hips. You may need a block.

1 Start in mountain pose.

2 On an exhalation, step your right foot out so that your feet are 110–140cm (3½–4½ feet) apart. Inhale, raise your arms up parallel to the floor and reach them out to the sides, keeping your arms straight and palms down.

3 Turn your left foot in slightly to the right so the foot is diagonal. Your right foot should be out, facing forwards and leading. Align the right heel with the left heel. Turn your right thigh outward, so that the right kneecap is in line with the centre of the right foot.

4 Keeping your left leg straight, exhale and bend your right knee over the right ankle at 90 degrees, keeping the shin perpendicular to the floor.

5 Bring your right hand down towards the outside of the right foot, either placing the right hand flat on the floor or on a block. Extend your left arm straight up towards the ceiling, then turn the left palm to face towards your head and reach the arm over the back of your left ear, palm facing the floor, bicep near your ear. Stretch from your left heel through your left fingertips trying to keep a straight line, lengthening the entire left side of your body. Look towards your left hand and try to open through the front of your body, holding the shape.

6 Remain in the posture for 5–10 breaths. Inhale to come up. Push both heels strongly into the floor and, using your core, come up.

7 Reverse the feet and repeat to the left side.

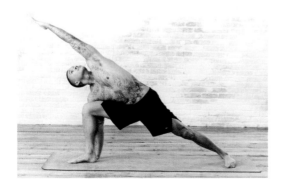

PARIVRTTA PARSVAKONASANA
REVOLVED SIDE ANGLE POSE

Good for stretching your spine, lower back, glutes and hips.

1 Start in mountain pose.

2 On an exhalation, step your left foot out so that your feet are 110–140cm (3½–4½ feet) apart. Inhale, raise your arms up parallel to the floor and reach them out to the sides, keeping your arms straight and palms down.

3 Turn your right foot in slightly to the left so the foot is diagonal. Your left foot should be out, facing forwards and leading. Align the left heel with the right heel. Turn your left thigh outward, so that the left kneecap is in line with the centre of the left foot.

4 Keeping your right leg straight, square your hips, turning your torso to the left. Then twist your hips and start to bring your right elbow over your left thigh, trying to bring your armpit into the thigh. Bend your left knee over the left ankle at 90 degrees keeping the shin perpendicular to the floor. Place your

hands into a prayer position, palms together, and twist your body, looking towards the ceiling. Suck your stomach in and keep twisting through every breath.

5 Remain in this pose for 5–10 long breaths. Exhale, release the twist and bring your torso back to upright with an inhalation to standing.

6 Repeat the same steps for the other side.

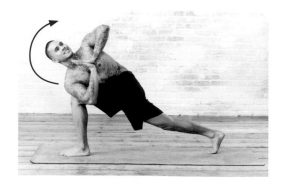

PARSVOTTANASANA
PYRAMID POSE

Good for stretching your shoulders, forearms, chest, hamstrings and hips.

1 Start in mountain pose.

2 On an exhalation, step your right foot out so that your feet are 110–140cm (3½–4½ feet) apart. Inhale, raise your arms up parallel to the floor and reach them out to the sides, keeping your arms straight and palms down.

3 Turn your left foot in slightly to the right so the foot is diagonal. Your right foot should be out, facing forwards and leading. Align the right heel with the left heel. Turn your right thigh outward, so that the right kneecap is in line with the centre of the right foot.

4 Exhale and rotate your torso to the right, squaring the front of your pelvis. Then bring your hands behind your back and put your hands together in reverse prayer. Try and squeeze your elbows back and squeeze your palms together. Suck your belly in and open your chest on an inhale.

5 Exhale and start leaning your torso over the right leg. Make sure you keep your hips as straight as you can. Press the thighs back and lengthen the torso forward, lifting through the top of the sternum. Keep your legs as straight as you can. If you are not very flexible, just bring your torso towards your leg as far as you can. If you're more flexible, bring your head towards your shin or knee.

6 Hold this posture for 5–10 long breaths then come up with an inhalation by pressing actively through the back heel, using your core.

7 Then go to the left side.

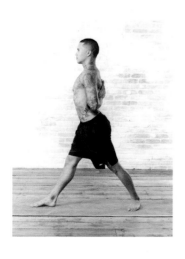
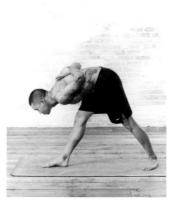

DANDASANA
STAFF POSE

This is a warm-up for your spine and hips before you do the Paschimottanasana opposite. You may need 2 blocks.

1 Sit on the floor with your legs together straight out in front of you. If your torso is leaning back it might be better to sit on a blanket, block or a bolster to lift the pelvis. When you're in this position, your torso should be as straight as possible.

2 Keep your shoulder blades back, lift the chest and bring your chin slightly down.

3 Flex your ankles and place your hands on the floor, with straight arms by your sides. Push through your hands.

4 Now push your torso away from the floor (or on blocks), imagine elongating your spine, sucking your belly in – lengthen as much as you can.

5 Stay here for 5 long deep breaths. Remain seated on the floor.

PASCHIMOTTANASANA A & B
SEATED FORWARD BEND

Good for stretching your hamstrings, calves, hips and lower back. You may need a strap and/or a block.

1 Sit on the floor with your legs together straight out in front of you. If your torso is leaning back, it might be better to sit on a blanket, block or a bolster to lift the pelvis. When you're in this position, your torso should be as straight as possible.

2 Suck your belly in and lift your chest open on an inhale then start to fold forward on an exhale, bringing your torso over your thighs and legs. Use a strap if you have tight hamstrings – place it around your feet and move your grip forward each side until you feel the stretch. If you're more flexible you can grab your big toes with your two forefingers and thumbs.

3 Fold forward as much as you can, keeping your back as straight as possible and looking towards your feet. Push your knees down towards the floor, straightening your legs. Pull from your hands and arms, keeping your elbows out to the sides and relaxing your shoulders.

4 Stay here for 5 deep breaths.

5 After you've done this, you can try this Paschimottanasana B for a deeper variation. Lift your head and torso, inhale and open your chest. If using a strap, bring your hands in closer to your feet, otherwise bring your hands around the sides of your feet. If you are more flexible, you can bind your fingers together or grab your wrists.

6 Fold forward, this time bringing your head onto your legs, and relax. If using a strap, keep your head up and keep looking at your feet.

7 Stay here for 5 long deep breaths then release. Remain seated.

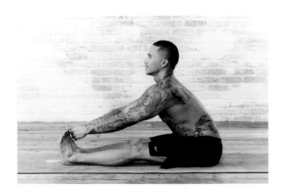
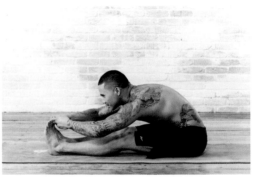

JANU SIRSASANA A
HEAD TO KNEE POSE

Good for stretching your hips, lower back, hamstrings and calves.

1 Sit on the floor with your left leg straight out in front of you, with the foot flexed towards you. Bend your right knee out to the side, and draw the heel of your right foot towards your perineum, placing the sole of your foot on the inside of the left inner thigh.

2 Turn your torso slightly to the left, keeping your hips as square as possible, then lifting the torso on the inhale, sucking your belly in, fold forward over your left leg on an exhale.

3 Holding either the ankle or around the foot, keeping your belly sucked in, bring your stomach towards the thigh, pulling towards your ankle.

4 Bring your chin towards your shin and look down towards your leg.

5 Stay here for 5 breaths, inhale and lift the chest, and then repeat on the other side.

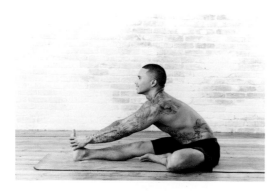
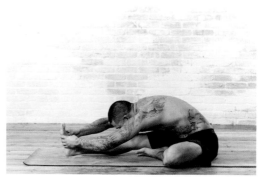

MARICHYASANA A

Good for stretching hips, hamstrings, shoulders and back. You may need a block to sit on.

1 Sit on the floor with your left leg straight out in front of you, flexing the foot towards you. Bend your right knee up to the ceiling with the foot flat on the floor, about one hand space away from your left leg. Try to bring the right heel as close to your right glute as possible.

2 Inhale, lift your torso and begin to wrap your right arm around your right leg, rotating the arm inwards. Try to get your shin into the armpit. Sweep the forearm around the outside of the leg. The right hand will press against the outside of the left thigh or glute.

3 Bring the left arm around behind your back. Clasp the left wrist in the right hand, if you are flexible enough, otherwise hold your fingers. Then exhale and extend your torso forward. Relax your shoulders and draw them away from your ears, draw the shoulder blades actively down your back.

4 Stay in position for 5 long breaths, then come up as you inhale. Repeat on the other side for the same length of time.

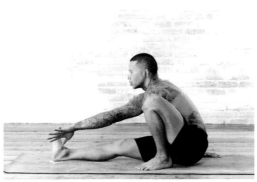
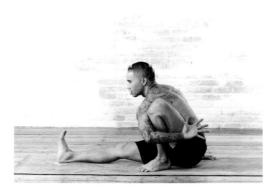
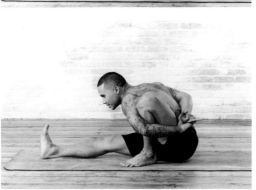

BADDHA KONASANA
BUTTERFLY POSE

Good for stretching your hips, groin and lower back. You may need a block or a bolster.

1 Sit with your legs out in front of you with your legs slightly bent. Sit on a block or bolster if your hips feel tight. Bend your knees, bring the soles of your feet together and bring your heels close to your groin, allowing your knees to go out to the sides.

2 Grab the insides and outsides of your feet with your forefingers and thumbs and open your feet like a book, keeping the edges of the feet on the floor.

3 Make sure you are sitting up straight and tall. Don't force your knees down.

4 Stay in this pose anywhere from 1 to 2 minutes. Try not to force the stretch, but try to relax into it through controlled, slow breathing. Then inhale, lift your knees away from the floor and extend the legs back to their original position.

5 For a harder variation, open the feet up like a book and begin to bring the head down towards the feet, going as deep as you comfortably can. Stay there for 1 to 2 minutes, relaxing into the pose.

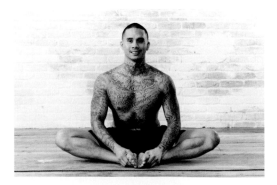
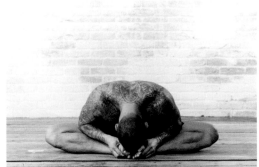

SUPTA PADANGUSTHASANA A & B
RECLINING HAND TO BIG TOE POSE

Good for stretching your hips and hamstrings. You may need a strap.

1 Lie on your back, with both legs extended out in front of you.

2 Slowly raise the right leg straight up and hold the big toe of the right foot with the two forefingers and thumb of the right hand. If you have tight hamstrings you can loop a strap around the arch of the right foot and hold the strap in both hands.

3 Inhale and straighten the knee and leg, pressing the right heel up towards the ceiling, and pull your toe towards you. If using a strap you can walk your hands up the strap until the elbows are fully extended. Keeping the hands as high on the strap as possible.

4 Begin with the raised leg perpendicular to the floor. Bring your left hand over your left thigh and push down. If you can lift your head, bring it to your right knee and hold. If you cannot do this then you can just rest your head on the floor.

5 Stay here for 5–10 long breaths, keeping your legs straight.

6 Then while pushing your left hand down onto your left thigh, bring your right leg out to the right, towards the floor, keeping your legs as straight as you can. Make sure your hips are square and your glutes are both on the floor. Bring the right leg as close to the floor as you can. Look over your left shoulder and stay here for 5–10 long breaths.

7 Bring the right leg back to the centre of the body and release your hold. Repeat on the left side.

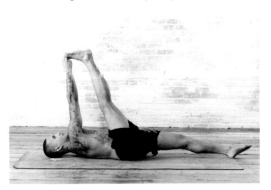

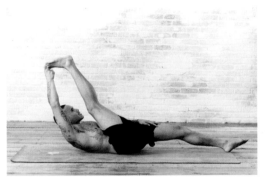

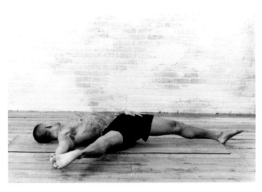

SETU BANDHASANA AND URDHVA DHANURASANA
BRIDGE AND FULL WHEEL

Step 1 is Setu Bandhasana. All 4 steps make up the Full Wheel.

Good for stretching your shoulders, spine and chest.

1 For the Setu Bandhasana and the first step of the Full Wheel, lie on your back, arms by your sides, knees above your heels, feet parallel and hip width apart. Lift your bum in the air and push through your hips using your legs. Interlace your fingers under your bum and straighten your arms. Wiggle your shoulders to open up the chest as much as you can, keep pushing your hips up – see first picture below. Stay here for 5 breaths then come back down the mat and relax.

2 Keep your feet where they are. Bring your hands behind your ears, inverting your hands down towards the floor, fingers pointing towards your feet and elbows to the ceiling. Initially lift through your hips first, just a couple of inches and then slowly lift your shoulder blades and lower back simultaneously and use your legs to help push up. Now push through your arms, trying to straighten them, lifting your hips towards the ceiling. Really open through your chest and shoulders. At first you may not be able to straighten your arms or raise your hips; do what you can.

3 Stay here for 5 long breaths and then slowly come down, bringing your chin in to your chest as you come down. Then lie down and prepare to come up one more time.

4 Push up again in the same way. Step your feet closer to your hands to go deeper into this posture. If you don't feel you can, just stay where is good for you. Hold for 5 long deep breaths. It's really important to breathe deeply in this posture, it will help to relax and open you up. Then tuck your chin, bend your elbows (keeping them shoulder width apart), and lower back down to the mat.

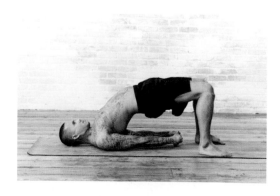
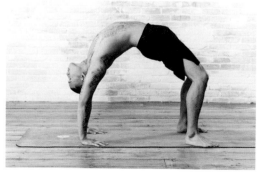

EKA PADA RAJAKAPOTASANA
MERMAID POSE

Good for stretching your quads, hip flexor and shoulders. You may need a strap and/or a cushion.

1 Begin on all fours, with your knees directly below your hips. Bring your hands up off the ground and straighten up on to your knees. Bring your right knee forward to 90 degrees in front of you, with your right foot flat on the floor. Make sure your right foot is in front of your left knee (which is on the floor). The right knee can angle slightly to the right, outside the line of the hip. Keep your hips as square as you can.

2 Bring your left foot off the floor and try and grab your left foot with your left hand. If you cannot reach then use a strap around the foot. Pull the foot towards your left glute and push both hips forward opening through your hips. If you experience pain in your knee, place a cushion underneath or fold over your mat for more padding. Rest your right hand on your right knee for stability.

3 If you can maintain the upright position, and you feel that you can stretch more, then bring your right hand back to grab the foot as well. Lift through your chest, push forward through your hips. Try to keep your hips square and elongate through your spine.

4 Hold for 5 long breaths. From this position, if you're more flexible and can go deeper into the posture then slide the top of your foot down the inside of your left arm until it reaches the crease of the elbow. If not, repeat Step 3 and bring the heel closer to your bum.

5 Then bring your left hand towards the back of your head and try and grab the left hand with your right hand, binding behind your head. Your right elbow should be pointing up towards the ceiling.

6 Try to push your left hip forwards, opening your chest, and lean through your hips. Stay here for 5 long deep breaths and then release the bind and slowly come out of the posture.

7 Repeat on the other side.

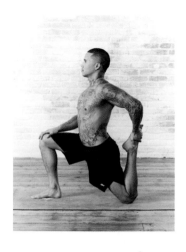
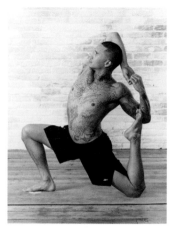

SIRSASANA
HEADSTAND

This is called the king of all poses and it will take time to get right. If you feel pain in your neck or head, stick with the first stage. Use the wall and make sure the surrounding space is safe for practice.

1 Kneel on the floor, interlace your fingers and set the forearms down on the floor, elbows at shoulder width. Now from here, place the crown of your head onto the floor and hug your hands into the back of the head. Make sure your hands are wrapped tightly to the back of the head and you are not resting on your forehead or the back of your head.

2 Tuck your toes under and lift your knees off the mat. Press your hands and elbows down to the floor really using your shoulders and arms to push away. This will take the pressure away from your head. Now walk your feet towards your hands, keeping your legs as straight as you can. Stay here for 5 deep breaths. Practise until this is comfortable, then you can move to the next stage.

3 From here, walk your feet in until all the weight is in your arms and shoulders, then bring one foot away from the floor. Bring your heel to your bum, then, leaning forward, you can bring the other heel to your bum and balance here. Keep pressing down firmly through the floor and suck in your belly. You can try this by a wall for some extra support at first.

4 From here you can start to raise both legs together towards the ceiling at the same time. Continue to press the shoulder blades against the back and keep the weight evenly balanced on your two forearms while pushing away from the floor. Once the backs of the legs are fully lengthened and straight, maintain that length and point your toes.

5 Stay here for 10 seconds and gradually increase the time over the days and weeks. Then you can try it fully away from the wall, once you can find the balance without using the wall at all. The aim is to stay here for 25 long deep breaths. This is your long-term goal.

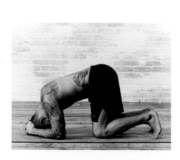
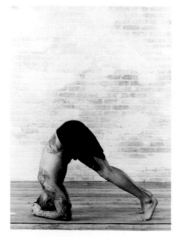
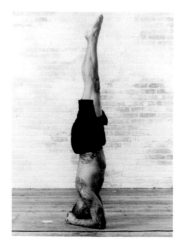

PADMASANA
LOTUS POSE

Good for stretching your hips.

1 Sit on the floor crossed leg. Bend your right knee and bring the lower leg up into a cradle then just rock your leg back and forth a few times, opening through your hip.

2 Then place the right foot on the left thigh, heel towards your hip and rest the right knee on the left foot. This is half padmasana (lotus). If your knee doesn't come down to the floor, sit on a block or a bolster and cross your legs in a comfortable position. If you can neither do this then just keep practising the cradle rocks.

3 Then, if you can, grab your left foot and place this foot on top of the right thigh. So both feet are resting on opposite thighs. You want to aim to get the foot towards the hips but this will only happen over time as you become more flexible. Be careful and stay aware of your knees. If you feel any pain then slowly take a few steps back and just stay there. Treat your knees like glass in this pose. Do not force yourself into the pose through pain.

4 Place the top of your hands on your knees, palms up, forefinger and thumb touching and the other three fingers straight (this is a mudra). Arms should be straight and chin slightly down. Stay here for 10 long deep breaths, filling your lungs with as much oxygen as you can, breathing in and out of the nose in a strong ujjayi breath. Once finished slowly come out of posture and lie down.

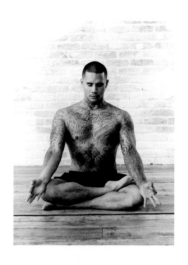 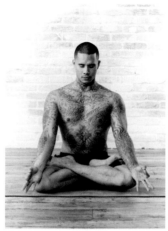

SAVASANA
CORPSE POSE

Good for relaxing and healing the body. The whole yoga practice has led to this finishing posture – the corpse pose – this is for all the energy you've created to be absorbed into the body and heal the internal organs, muscles and mind.

1 Lie on your back with your knees slightly bent to the side. Your feet should be slightly wider than hip width and your arms on the floor by your sides, palms facing upwards.

2 Keep your head centred, not allowing it to fall to either side.

3 Relax every part of your body and try to let go of any tension. Breathe normally and stop using ujjayi breath now.

4 Close your eyes and stay here for 3–10 minutes.

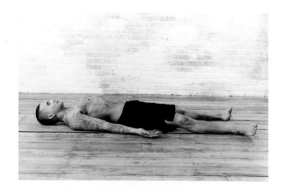

PRANAYAMA BREATH CONTROL

'Prana' means breath, life, energy or strength. 'Ayama' means stretch, extension, length or control. Patanjali, ancient sage and author of the Yoga Sutras, describes pranayama as the controlled intake and outflow of breath in a posture.

Pranayama is one of the eight limbs of yoga and is an important part of the practice. It is a form of meditation, and it also helps to relax our minds, brain and nervous system. Its main purpose is to help the respiratory system to function at its best and improve lung capacity. It's believed it can help to purify the body, mind and intellect.

Sit in padmasana or half padmasana (page 207), sitting on a block if you need to. Keep your torso active and allow your arms and legs to be relaxed as if you were sleeping. Keep the chin slightly down. You can close your eyes keeping your vision inward towards your third eye chakra.

Do this before meditation or when you feel anxious; it even helps to strengthen your lungs. It can complement your training programme whenever you feel you need to take time for you.

SAMA VRITTI PRANAYAMA

Start with this before doing nadi shodhana below.

1 Sit in padmasana (page 207), half padmasana or just with crossed legs. Sit on a block if you need to.

2 Keep your hands by your knees or in a mudra (page 27) on your knees.

3 Start with an inhale through the nose for 3–5 seconds and then exhale through the nose for the same duration. Make sure you have a perfect soft, smooth rhythm.

4 Once you feel comfortable with this you can attempt to hold your breath after the inhalation, first for a few seconds. Exhale and repeat, back to an inhale again for the same length, then hold, etc.

5 Keep the inhalation and exhalation always at the same length, over time increase the length of time you hold your breath for, until you can reach the same time for inhalation, hold and exhalation.

6 Do this for 5–6 rounds.

NADI SHODHANA (ALTERNATE NOSTRIL BREATHING)

Do this once or twice a week in conjunction with sama vritti. Only start this pranayama after you have completed a couple of weeks of sama vritti pranayama alone.

1 Bend your two forefingers closed and stick out your thumb and your last two fingers including the pinky finger.

2 Gently exhale and fully close your right nostril with your thumb, placing it just under the bone. Inhale through your left nostril, maintaining an even flow of breath. Keep the breath soft, slow and smooth and when you breathe in, fill the lungs all the way, as much as you can.

3 When your lungs are full, block the left nostril with your pinky and second last finger, hold the breath for a second, and prepare and adjust your fingers for exhalation.

4 Exhale though the right nostril, synchronizing the exhale of breath with the extension and expansion of the ribs. This is one round. Repeat these rounds first, five times.

5 Finish on the same nostril as you started. Slowly work up to doing this for up to 5 minutes.

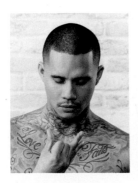 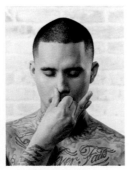 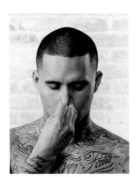 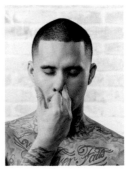

MEDITATION

Meditation has many benefits: the reduction of stress, the ability to control anxiety, a greater perspective, increased self-awareness and improved mental clarity, focus and concentration.

I try to meditate every day. It has helped me get through stressful, emotional times. It also helps me to live in the present moment without worrying about any stresses or issues that are going on in the outside world.

When you first start with meditation it might feel quite hard. The only way to get better at meditation is to practise it consistently and frequently. When you do this meditation, first start by challenging yourself to a few minutes, say 3–5 minutes, and then slowly start increasing this by one minute each day until you reach 10 minutes or more.

I'm going to teach you a meditation where we concentrate on the breath. You can do it by sitting down crossed leg on the floor, in padmasana (or half padmasana) or simply lying down. Keep your back straight and hands on your knees or in a mudra. Sit on a block if you need to.

The simplest way to get into the meditative state is to begin by listening and relaxing.

1 Close your eyes and allow yourself to be aware. Hear all the sounds that are going on around you. Don't try to identify these sounds by listening to what it exactly is, just hear the sounds for what they are. Just allow the sound to be a sound. Take a moment here to get into this state.

2 Once you have been able to relax and allow the sounds to be just sounds, I want you to start slowly concentrating on your breath. Breathing normally and freely in and out through your nose, let your breath just be itself don't try and force any type of particular breathing just as when you're breathing and you don't realize. Relax your body, face and any other parts of your body. Then all I want you to do is simply observe your breath. Just watch every inhalation and every exhalation that goes in and out through your nose. I just want you to witness the rhythm, and the motion of the breath and focus all of your attention on your breathing. Don't worry about anything else going on around you or in your life, allow all your focus to be on your breath. Take a few moments here to get into this state.

3 What you will have noticed when concentrating and observing the breath is your mind starting to think about different thoughts, thoughts coming into your mind and leaving, then another thought entering your mind then leaving. Now what I want you to do is to just allow these thoughts to take place. A lot of thoughts run through your mind – don't try to block any of these thoughts out. Allow your mind to be free but as soon as you realize that you're thinking about these thoughts then I want you to bring your attention and your concentration back to your breath, back to observing the inhalation and exhalation. This is meditation.

4 Stay here and do this firstly for 3–5 minutes then slowly work your way up to 10 minutes or longer.

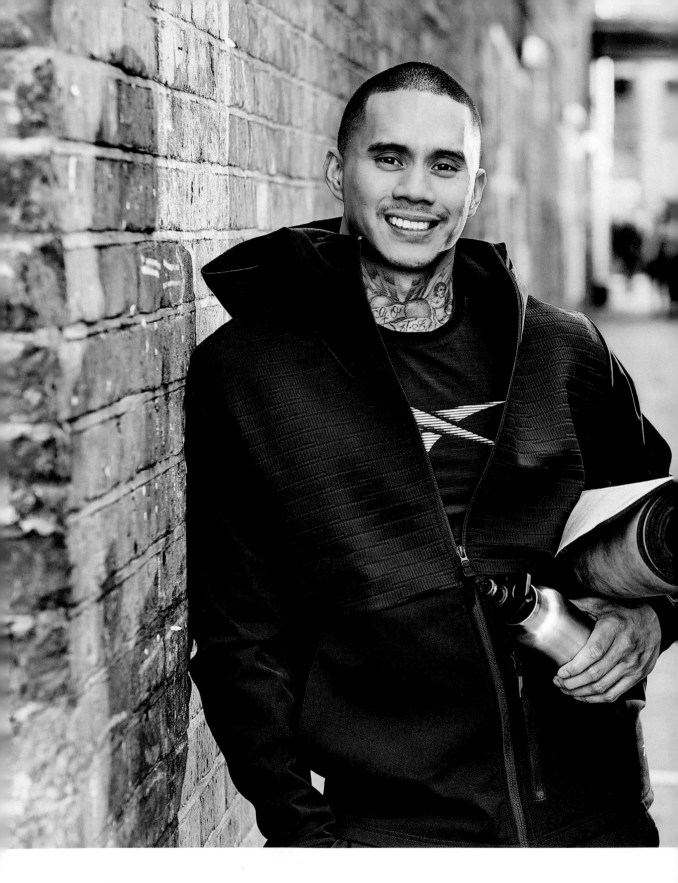

4

BE THE FITTEST

Allow yourself to have a little bit of whatever you consider a treat – relax your diet a little, for example – but try to maintain a balance.

Well done on completing your first Be The Fittest three-month programme! I hope you found it challenging, but that you enjoyed it and hopefully learnt some new things along the way.

What next?

In this section I'm going to help you understand how to maintain your progression, and also how to create new goals to keep happy and motivated and remain in focus. I'm going to teach you how to manipulate your programme to make it your own, so that you can work on your individual strengths and weaknesses.

Recovery and time off

Taking time off is a very important part of your fitness life. It is going to help you to achieve your goals. Training every day with the same intensity, day after day, with no break can be detrimental.

So after you've completed your three-month programme, take one or two weeks off. You don't have to rest completely but I'd like you to do something totally different, whether that's playing a new sport or taking up something else that still requires you to be active. Just make sure you're not doing the same thing that you've been doing during the last three months. You can be as creative as you want, make sure you use this time to enjoy yourself.

Also allow yourself to have a little bit of whatever you consider a treat – relax your diet a little, but at the same time I still want you to try to maintain a balance.

I would recommend taking two weeks off but if you really want to, you can do another programme after a minimum one-week break.

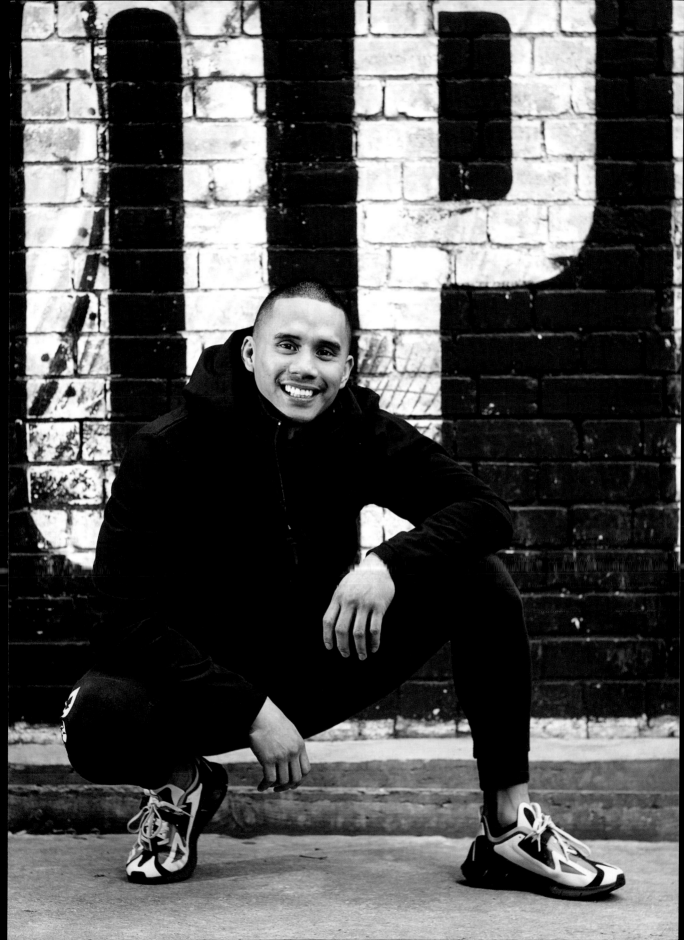

RECOVERY AND SELF-CARE

1 ▶ Foam roller and trigger point massage ball
Using a foam roller and a trigger point massage ball is one of the best and greatest ways to help loosen any tight muscles and to relieve any trigger points in your body. These also help when I feel like I've strained muscles and will help to speed up recovery from injuries or niggles. The foam roller can be used on larger body parts like your quadriceps or your calf muscles. Use the trigger point ball to work on smaller body parts – your glutes, your rotator cuff, forearms and hips.

2 ▶ Sports massage
A sports massage is great way to relieve your body and your muscles from a hard training session and soothe any aches and pains. It's one of the most effective ways to help the body to recover.

3 ▶ A hot Epsom salts bath
A nice hot bath can penetrate your muscles and help them to recover from a hard training session – adding in Epsom salts can help to reduce inflammation and soreness.

4 ▶ Nutrition
Make sure you stick to the diet, keeping to a balanced plan, and make sure you take your vitamins. If you feel like you're lacking in energy, add a little bit more carbohydrate into your system. Nutrition is a key factor in your body's recovery.

5 ▶ Sleep
Make sure you get enough sleep. Try not to look at your phone or be too active an hour before bedtime. Having a great sleep will help you to wake up fresh the next day.

6 ▶ Meditation
Meditation helps to train the mind and bring clarity. Do it consistently and you will reap the benefits – see also page 211.

7 ▶ Daily gratitude
It's important to give thanks for your blessings – for all the good things that have come to you in your life. Take a little time every day to remember how fortunate you are and the times you've enjoyed, especially when you're stressed or feeling down. It can help just to stop and think that a situation could be worse.

8 ▶ Breathwork
Breathing is much more than just an involuntary process, as you'll learn when you practise the exercises on pages 209–210. Breathing mindfully and deliberately is invaluable in helping you control your anxiety and relieve stress. It's ideal before meditation to help you begin with a calm mind and it can help to build up lung strength.

9 ▶ Do what you enjoy
It might sound obvious, but take time to do things that you enjoy, whether that's a hobby, socializing with friends – or whatever makes you happy and makes you laugh. I find this is so important for self-care and for your mental health.

STAYING MOTIVATED

Following a programme for three months can be really tough. Sometimes you can get distracted and at times certain situations in your life can lead you to become demotivated. This little section is here to help you to get through any types of motivation loss and aid with regaining your focus and mental clarity.

Remember that training isn't easy. Following a diet isn't easy. If these things were easy, then everyone would be the fittest person on earth and everyone would look amazing. Over the years of training and the time I've spent with my clients, one of the most common things I have seen that stops people from achieving their goals is not being able to find that self-discipline to get up in the morning and stay focused enough to follow the plan and exercise accordingly.

You have to dig deep inside yourself and ask yourself why you're reading this book; question why you haven't achieved these goals so far. You have to change something about yourself in order to change the results ahead.

You also have to understand that not every single session is going to be an amazing one. Some sessions you have will be good, other sessions might be terrible, but they go hand in hand. Try not to become attached to having an amazing session each time, because your expectations will be too high.

If you do have a bad session or even if your session just doesn't feel as great as the one before, take it with a pinch of salt, and accept it for what it is. The most important thing is being consistent: making sure you get your sessions in, trying and giving your best 100% of the time.

I have bad sessions myself sometimes. I work with Olympic athletes, and even they have bad sessions sometime. You have to take the rough with the smooth and just always remember why you are here and what we are trying to achieve. Make sure that you're not going to let anything stop you from reaching that goal. It's all about self-discipline and it's all in your mind.

I know that anyone who is reading this book is capable of amazing things. You can achieve anything you put your mind to, so stay with it, keep training hard, always give 100% and keep spreading great energy.

MY KEY TIPS

1 ▶ Monitor those your goals. Remember those goals you listed on page 12? Any time you feel demotivated, look back at where you started and compare it with what you have achieved. Look at where you want to be and get that fire back in your belly.

2 ▶ Find friends or family who have the same mindset as you who are also trying to achieve their goals. It really helps to share stories and experiences and to have someone to talk to when you're feeling demotivated. They can help to pick you up and vice versa.

3 ▶ Find a good playlist. I always find music helps me get through a workout and helps me to push through when I feel I'm running out of energy or I can't do it any more. Create your own playlists that you can look forward to working out to, or you can follow my playlists through my social media accounts.

4 ▶ Think twice when you're in the kitchen. When you feel tempted to eat something that you're not supposed to or you feel you might be about to throw your day out of the window, always think twice. Go back to why you're doing this, what you're trying to achieve and remember everything that goes into your stomach will either help you, or not, to achieve your goals.

5 ▶ Enjoy it and have fun! Health and fitness should be fun and you should always look forward to it. Sometimes it might be a gruelling hard session and you might be hating it at the time, afterwards I want you to feel relieved and be like, 'Do you know what, I enjoyed that pain in a strange way!'. The reason I've been doing what I do for years is because I enjoy it and I have fun. I want you guys to feel the same way! For me training and fitness is always going to be a part of my life because I love what I do 100%.

Creating new goals

So, having completed this three-month programme you will have probably found a lot of it quite tough. For those of who you feel like you haven't achieved anything, remember we are always trying to improve and move to the next level and learn more.

I know that there will be parts of the programme that you have struggled with or that you found tough and what I want you to do is to create some new goals. Sit down and think about furthering your skill assets, improving your strength and your fitness, and working on your weaknesses.

Have a think about what you struggled with or what you feel are your weaknesses and write down your top five new goals that you want to achieve. Some can be long-term, some can be short-term. When you create your new programme I want you to have these goals as your objectives.

MAKE THIS YOUR OWN

Once you have created your new goals, I want you to follow this programme again but implementing your new goals into it. I also want you to keep working on your weaknesses, specifically on the exercises that you struggle with to always ensure you're improving. Make sure you add 3 sets of 10–15 reps of those exercises that you struggle with during your Work on your Weaknesses days; do this over a period of a month. After one month if you feel that you're able to do these exercises sufficiently well then over the next month, work on a new set of exercises that need improvement.

For this new programme, I want you to replace one of the workouts each week with one that relates specifically to your new goals; so for instance if you wanted to be more flexible or work more on wellbeing then can replace an exercise workout with a yoga practice, or add more meditation to it.

If you wanted to work more on lower body strength, you could replace an upper body workout with a lower body one.

You can apply this customization to any goal you strive for, whether it's a single goal or a few goals. Just write them down and then add whichever workouts and exercises will help with achieving these.

All I want you to do is stick to the ground rules and foundation I've outlined in the book, but now you can make your own programme. Remember to make it feasible and something that you know you can achieve and stick to for 3 months.

Keep me posted

I want all of you to achieve amazing results. I want all of you to get to a point in life in which you're able to change your mindset, health and fitness to live a better, happy, healthier life. Nothing would make me happier than for you to keep me updated with your workouts and all your progress. Post on your social media and use #bethefittest

Feel free to hit me up and I'll do my very best to get back to you!

INDEX

ACKNOWLEDGEMENTS

Firstly, I'd like to thank God for every blessing in my life and every test, and for giving me the strength to be where I am in life. Gem, my beautiful soulmate, wifey, best mother to all my kids – since the age of 15 you have been in my life, you have seen me at my lowest and helped me when I failed, been there through thick and thin. You are the best mother in the world to my kids and without you I would not be where I am nor would I be able to do what I do. I know I don't thank you enough so I'd like to dedicate this to you by saying thank you and I love you. I'd like to thank my kids – Taleah, you're the reason I started my business, I love you; Olivia and River, you both give me so much joy and keep me striving to succeed more to make your lives better than I had it. I'd like to thank my mother and my sister for everything you did for me when I was growing up and my stepdad for helping me all the times I needed you. My mum, Clive and sister: love you always.

I'd like to thank Sean and Geraldine for helping me during the hard times, for always being there for me and my kids, for always having your door open, and being like parents.

I'd like to thank all my friends and family. To my cuzzy Karen for giving me my first yoga book when my life was in trauma. Shout man like Dash, Scardey, Clem, LA, Supa, pringle and all the man dem, you know who you are, so many names to mention. Always been there from a young age, my Day Ones. Thank you to GI Joe for showing me the way in personal training – you inspired me, brother. My brother Karlтом – thank you, bro, for those training sessions and the callisthenics in Battersea, we learnt a lot.

I'd also like to thank everyone at The Prince's Trust for being an amazing charity, helping me and thousands of others to start businesses. Nick Hynes, you have been an amazing mentor – thank you for always believing in me and all your words are gold dust. Neil Mahoney from the Trust – thank you. You have always believed in me and always had time for me. I appreciate all the opportunities you put me forward for. Danny Richman, best SEO workshops ever! Words of gold dust. Susan Glenn – thank you for being my first mentor, you always believed in me and still check up on me and I am grateful to you and your husband for everything! Thank you to Jo Chin for great advice and support.

Thank you to all my yoga teachers – Stewart Gilchrist, Ryan Spielman, Emi Tull, Mark Kan. I'd also like to shout triyoga – best yoga centre, first place I ever tried and have always supported, thank you Genny. All of you – thank you for all your knowledge and the time you have spent

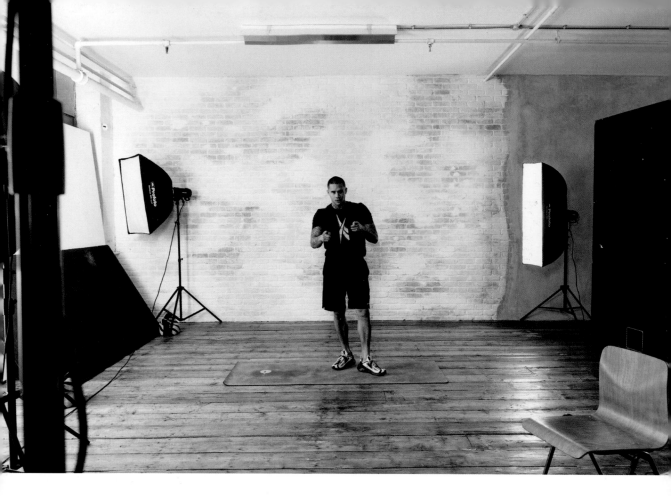

with me. Thank you to everyone at Reebok and Grenade for believing in me and supporting me.

Thank you to my clients – all of you have been great; a lot of laughs, tears and hard work but we got results. You guys inspire me; thanks for being patient with me. Thank you to Ellen, Nadia and Gemma at Mokkingbird talent management and Lauren Gardner at Bell Lomax Moreton for believing in me and for everything you've done. Thank you to the team at Quadrille for believing in me and giving me this opportunity. Massive thank you to Scot Paterson who helped me create lots of the recipes in the book, and dieticians 'Today with Rosé' who helped sign off our recipes and tweak them so they could be the healthiest and most balanced. Thank you to every supporter of mine – you guys give me the inspiration to keep me doing what I do. Keep supporting me and spread the word. Shout to anyone I have not mentioned here but talk and speak to on a regular!

And a massive thank you to all of you out there who support everything I do, all my members on Workout with Ty, everyone who follows and supports me on my socials and you guys who have bought this book! Thank you from the bottom of my heart and keep supporting. Love you all!